The Safe Child

RICHARD C. GOSSAGE

How to encourage

safety awareness

in your child or teenager

KEY PORTER BOOKS

Canadian Cataloguing in Publication Data

Gossage, Richard C.
    The safe child : how to encourage safety awareness in your child or
    teenager

ISBN 1-55013-919-3

1. Child rearing. 2. Safety education. I. Title.

HQ770.7G673   1997   649'.6   C97-932036-4

The publisher gratefully acknowledges the support of the Canada Council for the Arts and the Ontario Arts Council for its publishing program.

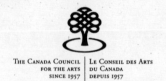

THE CANADA COUNCIL | LE CONSEIL DES ARTS
FOR THE ARTS | DU CANADA
SINCE 1957 | DEPUIS 1957

Key Porter Books Limited
70 The Esplanade
Toronto, Ontario
Canada M5E 1R2

Design: Jean Lightfoot Peters
Electronic formatting: Rena Potter
Illustrations: Kathryn Adams/3 in a Box

Printed and bound in Canada

97 98 99 00 6 5 4 3 2 1

The
Safe
Child

Contents

A Note from the Author

This is the third time in my life that I have tried to sit down and distill some thoughts that I hoped could help parents and other caregivers make life safer for their children as they grow up. For the last fifteen years, since my original effort with Mel Gunton, I have been continually involved with the subject. The good news is that I have been exposed to a great number of ideas. The bad news is that I can't possibly remember whether I thought them up or whether they came through reading and/or conversation with other experts. To those who see their ideas in my writing and who are not credited, I apologize. I hope I have done them justice. This book also contains elements from the 1982 effort which I feel have stood the test of time.

The majority of the book is a well-aged philosophy supported by lists of practical ideas which I strongly believe will equip you to give your children the best possible chance of growing up with less risk. However, I know that if you've picked up this book, you are already a concerned adult who is committed to child safety. As a result, I ask you to pass on those ideas that you believe are worthwhile to others who might benefit. If you do that, and get involved in excellent groups such as Block Parents, who have made child safety their crusade for over thirty years, then you can make a real difference. Only when we feel a responsibility for all children, rather than just our own, will childhood become safer for everyone!

Once again, I must credit Anna Porter, who persuaded me to take the plunge "just one more time." Also my appreciation goes to Susan Renouf, who pressured me gracefully, and to my editor, Barbara Tessman, who edited the manuscript so that I was hardly aware of what was hers and what was mine.

My sincere thanks to my assistant, Julie Leighton, who aided and abetted Susan by keeping me focused on the deadline and sane with fresh cups of tea, and made useful suggestions when she noticed inconsistencies as she processed the manuscript.

Finally, writing a book in your "free" time at the end of the working day and on weekends puts an inevitable and endless strain on your home life. It could not have happened without the steadfast support of my wife, Mary Lou, and my four children, Patrick, Caitlin, Tory, and Stephanie. May the four of you be as lucky with your children as Mary Lou and I have been with you!

A Word from the Block Parent Program of Canada

The Block Parent Program of Canada believes that education is the first step to safety. If a child is distressed and acts from knowledge, and not fear, he or she is more likely to be able to react safely to a potentially dangerous situation.

The Safe Child provides a great deal of information that we hope parents will use to educate their children so they can become confident individuals, thus enhancing their personal safety.

Block Parent Program of Canada

Introduction

Giving your children the knowledge and practical skills they need to look after themselves is as important as teaching them to read and write. Few parents or caregivers would disagree with this statement. Yet it's clear that, with greater effort, we could all do a better job in preparing our children to take care of themselves.

As adults, we can occasionally get away with being less than perfect in many aspects of our lives and relationships. It's not that we mean to be careless, it's just that we get tired or distracted and we slip up. Usually the slip goes unnoticed, but if we are caught we accept the responsibility, fix the problem, and get on with our lives. When it comes to our children's safety, however, we need to be reminded that, if we slip up, we may have to confront consequences few of us could bear.

In 1982, I co-authored a book entitled *A Parent's Guide to Streetproofing Children*. That book coined the word *streetproofing* and helped to focus attention on child safety. Since that time, I have been almost continuously involved with the issue. I have talked with numerous professionals, and seen lots of books, videos, games, and other products devoted to the topic. While parents and caregivers today have a huge array of materials offering advice, sometimes these materials give conflicting or erroneous suggestions.

I am not surprised when I hear that parents are confused and somewhat intimidated by the subject of child safety. It's hard to know where to start. You must make a conscious effort to search out the information, absorb it, and then determine whether or not it will work for your family.

When I say "work for your family," I mean: Are the suggestions something that you and your family can practice together? Is the advice something that you're actually going to follow? Wrapping your children in cotton batting and keeping them under guard on a remote island may guarantee their safety, but it's hardly practical. While that example is ludicrous, it makes the point that if you can't or won't follow the advice, then there isn't a chance that it will help keep your children safe, even if it sounds good in theory.

So when you consider advice for both you and your children, make sure that you agree with it. Ask yourself whether it makes sense, or whether it's a nice but ineffective cliché like "Don't talk to strangers."

Let's examine the value of that oddly enduring piece of advice. The strongest teacher is example, and we can't go through a day, unless it's on that guarded island, without talking to strangers. We talk to the stranger who rings up our purchases at the grocery store. We talk to the stranger who gases up our car at the service station. We teach our children to go to the door of a Block Parent, who may well be a stranger, when they feel threatened. If they go to a new school in the fall, they will be surrounded by children and teachers who are strangers. How can we ever explain all these exceptions?

Surely one of the most important skills that our children need to learn is how to meet and evaluate the personalities of new people—that is, *strangers*. How can they do this if they can't talk to them? Imagine if you kept your children on that mythical island until it was time for them to go to university, and then you dropped them off at the campus and said, "Have a great life!" You would be sending out the most vulnerable young adults that you could possibly have created. If ever there were marks who could be exploited by some unsavory individual, you've created them. If you want to help children be safe when they're older, you've got to let them meet and learn about others in controlled situations. The vast majority of people are kind, well-meaning individuals. "Don't talk to strangers" does not send that message.

Instead, such rules lead us to feel that we don't have any relationship with one another. When this happens, people will be less inclined to go to each other's aid. You don't have to be on intimate terms with the entire neighborhood, but if you stop and chat with individuals on the street or over the back fence when you're with your children, those youngsters are going to start to learn how other normal people behave. Only by understanding normal people do they have a chance of recognizing abnormal behavior if they do confront it.

That's not all. Odds are that if your child does have difficulty with another individual, that individual will be an acquaintance. So even if you could explain the "Don't talk to strangers" rule to your child, it could be dangerously misleading.

You may not agree with my feelings on strangers. That's perfectly all right. You are the person who knows what's best for your family, and ultimately it falls to you to keep them safe.

You should also know that, whatever your effort, tragedies can happen. Making your children safe is a function of playing the odds. The more you do right, the better their chances. Recent newspaper reports continue to reinforce that the defensive behaviors taught by various child-safety agencies do work. You must adopt a positive attitude, do the best that you can, and then hope and pray that your child will make it safely and securely to adulthood.

In this book, I'm going to illustrate the type of attitude that will help you keep your children safe. I will highlight areas of risk, and will include lots of practical ideas from sources in Canada, the United States, and England. My hope is that you will remember and use what you feel will work well for you.

Today, we are all far more conscious of the issue of child safety. The conviction of Graham James, the former hockey coach of the Swift Current Broncos, who pleaded guilty to two counts of sexually abusing young hockey players, and the trial of Francis Carl Roy, who is charged with the abduction and murder of Alison Parrott, have refocused the public's attention on the risks posed to children by sexual predators.

Those risks and issues relating to interaction with other people are still a parent's number one concern. A recent study by Milward Brown/ Abraxas Research for Stay Alert . . . Stay Safe looked into the priority that adult Canadians place on their children learning about abduction, bicycle safety, fire safety, road safety, and water safety. The study suggests that abduction (55 percent) outscores the other four threats (41 percent) combined in terms of being a priority concern in relation to children aged six to eleven. When the 15 percent who rated it their second-greatest concern are added, abduction climbs to a high of 70 percent. The findings of the study are largely unaffected by demographics, and it is interesting that abduction is the top concern whether or not the respondents have children of their own.

It is important to note, however, that such risks to children are far smaller than those posed by injury. It's a shocking fact that injuries are the leading cause of death in children and youth after their first year of life. Moreover, for every fatal injury, there are hundreds of non-fatal accidents that may result in long-term, or even permanent, functional disabilities.

Clearly, to have children you've got to be brave! On the positive side, you should know that, whatever you do, most children make it safely to adulthood. I am also convinced that the way you parent will be far more important than whether you remember a particular safety tip. As a result, this book will offer a number of parenting ideas that I hope will contribute to a safe childhood through a healthy parent–child relationship.

Chapter 1 Summary
A Philosophy for Improving the Odds

1. **Making children safe is hard work**
   ★ Don't be lazy.
   ★ Do everything in your power to eliminate potential hazards.

2. **Teach by example**
   ★ Children will do what you do, not what you say. Set an example on a continual basis.

3. **Role-play**
   ★ Create a role and situation to see how your children would behave. Refine your ideas together through creative play.

4. **Instill confidence in your children**
   ★ Making kids safe results largely from your efforts to make them believe in themselves and their ability to take responsibility for their own safety.
   ★ Provide information in a positive way: "Look both ways and you'll get across safely!"

5. **Make sure your communication is clear**
   ★ All discussions on safety should be two-way.
   ★ Describe the specific behavior you want changed.
   ★ Ask your children to tell you what you want them to do.

6. **Keep your children busy**
   ★ Get kids involved in their choice of activities when they are young.
   ★ Watching television is not an activity that can build their self-confidence.
   ★ Bored children might create their own activity, which could be dangerous.

7. **Safety is everyone's concern**
   ★ Use examples from the news to show that safety problems can affect everyone.

8. **Discipline**
   ★ As parents, if you simply trust your own judgment, and exercise your rights, you will go a long way toward helping your children.
   ★ Don't threaten and not follow through.
   ★ As a parent you have rights and should not be pushed around by your children.

9. **Children should earn their privileges**
   ★ Children who run into difficulties often have little sense of value.
   ★ Children who value their privileges are less likely to abuse them.

A Philosophy for Improving the Odds

Keeping your child safe takes hard work. It's just like anything else in life—if you want to be good, you're going to need to put in the time, all the time. In essence you've got to add a full-time job to the occupation that you already have, and that's tiring. How can you most effectively use your time to tilt the odds in favor of your children growing up both healthy and happy?

Making Children Safe Is Hard Work

The first point, which is often underemphasized, is that there are no halfway measures in terms of your child's safety. I'll give you a personal example of a situation that involved my daughter Caitlin.

The family was on holiday together. Caitlin was about eight or nine years old, bounding around in her bathing suit and bare feet. I was barbecuing hamburgers for lunch, and had used an electric barbecue-starter to fire up the coals. When they were well lit, I pulled out the red-hot starter and placed it carefully on a rock to cool off. It had been there for only about thirty seconds when Caitlin came around the corner of the cabin to see me. I was, of course, well aware of the danger and immediately admonished her to stay clear. No sooner had I finished my warning than she ran over to the lighter and jumped right on top of it. Her behavior was no different than if I'd instructed her to go and stand on the lighter. She let out the scream of a steer at roundup as the device branded the sole of her foot. I couldn't believe what had happened.

Later, after her recovery, she told me that she'd wanted to hop over the starter and had simply misgauged her jump. I asked her if she had heard me say that it was dangerous. "Oh yes!" she said. It seems that there was something about the danger that had actually attracted her. It was almost as if she would not have had the accident if I had said nothing. The real point, of course, is that I was lazy. I should have gone and picked up the starter or, at the very least, blocked her from going near it. Kids are unpredictable, and I was hoping that some words of advice would be enough. The message is that if you're aware of a potential hazard, do everything in your power to eliminate it.

Teach by Example

The next philosophical issue is that examples speak louder than words. This is something that we all know, but it means work, and sometimes we can all be lazy.

Having watched my own four children growing up, I've come to realize that they were like sponges absorbing what my wife, Mary Lou, and I did, whether or not we were consciously demonstrating something. I was driving my daughter Tory in the car when she was quite small. Suddenly she swore at a driver who had turned in front of me without signalling. Surprised, and slightly shocked, I asked her "Where did that come from?" She said, "Oh, that's what Mom says to bad drivers."

Mary Lou hadn't been trying to set an example in this way, but she had in any case.

The message is that you've got to plan to set an example on a continuous basis. Do up your seat belts when you get in the car. Look both ways before you cross the street. You may have observed out of the corner of your eye that there were no cars coming, but if your child does not see you looking up and down the street, she will think that you didn't bother to look.

Role-Play

Most children have great imaginations, and enjoy taking on the roles of others. One of the most effective ways I believe you can help your children learn about safety is by suggesting different situations and roles, and then letting them have some fun by showing you how they'd behave. It's an activity that can involve the whole family, and it gives you a chance to reinforce their correct behavior without giving them a lecture. The interaction will also get you thinking, and may help you refine some of your ideas so that they work better for your family.

Instill Confidence in Your Children

The third point is to do everything in your power to create a positive attitude in your children. Making them safe results, to a very large degree, from your efforts to make them believe in themselves and their ability to take responsibility for their own safety.

The problem is that the issue of child safety is very frightening for many adults. As a result, they tend to transmit that fear to their children. Child safety and streetproofing are about giving your children the confidence to know that they can eventually look after themselves when they are not in your care.

I'll give you an example from another area of risk—the water. All of us know that water can be very hazardous to our children. As a result, most of us enroll our children in swimming lessons at the earliest opportunity. Let's think about what happens in those lessons.

Generally, the instructor introduces the children to the new environment gradually in order to build their confidence. The class starts in the shallow end. The instructor dips each child's face into the water while the youngster is still standing so he or she can become accustomed to how it feels. The whole process revolves around tight control and building the children's confidence that they will be able to handle themselves in this new environment, if they trust the instructor and do what they are told.

Imagine if the instructor stood the children at the side of the pool and started off by stating, "If you don't move your hands and feet the way I tell you, you'll drown." You'll probably agree that it would be hard to get the children into the water after a statement like that. And yet that is very often the way in which we approach child safety.

Like all parents, mine used to shout at me when they saw me following a stray ball onto the street. "If you don't look both ways before you cross the street, you'll be hit by a car and killed," they would say. In essence, they thought they would help me by giving me a healthy fear of the street. As I got older, this strategy extended to other areas of the outdoors: "Don't walk through unlit parks at night in case you are attacked by a stranger." You already know what I think about the stranger issue; the point I want to make here is a different one. My parents could have provided the same information in a positive way. In the ball-chasing example, they could have said, "Look both ways before you cross the street to get your ball, and you'll get across safely." In terms of the park, more helpful advice would have been: "Take the well-lit streets on your way home instead of the short cut through the unlit park, and you're much less likely to be confronted by an unpleasant person."

A confident child is a safer child. Children who lack positive backing at home will unconsciously search it out elsewhere, and this makes them more vulnerable to gangs and cults on the street. Before recruiters will ask your child to join them, they will introduce themselves and generally be fairly open. They'll engage in conversation until they think the moment is right and then make the invitation. Another twist a recruiter might throw in is the observation "You look pretty down, and I know you don't know me, but if you want to grab a coffee I'm a good listener." Sound transparent and obvious? It is. But brought into play at the right time with the right kid, it can work. Remember, if a child feels alone and rejected or ignored at home, he is open to someone who claims to be willing to share his troubles. After all, no one is asking him to go to some out-of-the-way place; he's just being offered a coffee or a Coke and some conversation. What harm can that do?

Police agree that the majority of kids who get into trouble on the street do not like themselves. Whenever the police come into contact with the parents of kids who have had problems, the parents are always tremendously concerned. The police often wonder whether the problem might have been prevented if some of this concern had been turned into positive attention long before the crisis occurred.

A prime example of lack of a positive attitude is provided by Parents' Night at school. Those parents who turn up are always quick to ask the same question: "So what are the problems with my child?" Rarely do they ask what is going right, so they might return home and start by encouraging their children in those areas where they are doing well.

Social workers agree with the police that the kids who are most likely to get into trouble on the street are those who have a low opinion of themselves because they feel they are being ignored at home. One social worker described a conversation with a father whose daughter was in trouble. Although the man said that he spent a lot of time with his daughter, he could not remember when they'd last eaten a meal together. As the social worker stated, "If they dined together regularly, then maybe they'd start to talk." It's no use coming up to a child you haven't been around and saying, "So what's bugging you?"

Make Sure Your Communication Is Clear

That example leads nicely to the fourth big issue: you've got to make sure that your communication is clear. How many times have we told our children "Be careful!" What does that mean? If my daughter was riding her bicycle, and I said, "Be careful," did I mean that she should ride on the sidewalk? Was I telling her to stop at the stop signs?

The only way to know whether you are communicating effectively is to ask your children to tell you how they are supposed to change their specific behavior in response to what you've said. This will give you an indication of whether or not they understand. If they say they don't know what they should do, there is no point repeating the information in the same way. Failure to communicate is the fault of the speaker, so you have to be sure that the message is clear. Try to be more specific about what needs to be changed. "I want to see you wearing a bicycle helmet when you're on that bike so that you'll be protected if you ever fall off. Do you understand?" "Yes, Daddy! I mustn't go riding without my helmet." "Good, now get your helmet, and you can go and have some fun."

The corollary to making your communication clear is that all discussions on safety should be two-way. Now, I know that you're not going to have deep discussions with a toddler, but as your children get older, you should be asking their opinion on what they can do to stay safe in a particular situation. If you feel their answer is off base, ask them how they arrived at that conclusion. Rather than simply giving them the right answer, work with them to help them discover it themselves. If you've helped them to analyze the problem in their own minds, then you've greatly increased the odds that they will remember the issue and then act on it.

keep Your Children Busy

Your children are more likely to be safe if they are busy. My father used to say that his parents told him, "Idle hands are the devil's playground." I believe that there is more than a little homespun truth to that phrase. The problem is that, as a society, we've become very lazy. We consider children busy if they are watching television. Nothing could be further from the truth.

There are two very real difficulties with television. The first is program content. Much of it flies absolutely counter to any concept of child safety that you might reasonably be expected to hold. Individuals go down dark alleys; they fight back instead of getting out of the situation; and there are far more examples of bad guys leading abnormal lives than there are of good guys leading normal lives. Television is such a powerful medium that there are many books on this subject alone. You should read some of them, be aware of what your children are watching, and exercise appropriate influence.

The second difficulty is the actual construction of the programming. I believe that if a child is brought up with strong positive values, the content of television programming is less harmful than its overall structure. As you are probably aware, most television is packaged to sell advertising, which means that it tries to appeal to the broadest possible audience. If it's going to err, it will do so on the side of finding the lowest common denominator. Whether such packaging is the cause or the result of people having short attention spans doesn't matter. The point is that it reinforces the idea—particularly among children who spend a lot of time watching television—that if something isn't immediately interesting, it should change. This is further exaggerated by the ability to channel surf with a remote control.

Television is lowering children's boredom threshold far below that of previous generations. Today's children expect instant gratification, and that poses a parent some very real challenges. If children don't immediately understand or master something, they tend to define themselves as bored, and children who are bored are at greater risk of getting themselves into potentially dangerous situations.

To counteract this tendency, I believe that you should try to limit the amount of television that your children watch. In our family we do this by a simple rule—no television on school nights. This also has the benefit of encouraging children to take up other activities that expand their attention span. Those activities could range from reading to ballet to building models. The important thing is that your children learn to discover the joys of getting beyond the superficial and into the real world, where things aren't always perfect and may not always work the first time. Children who are busy with a variety of activities don't have as much opportunity to become bored.

I don't believe that children can be classified as good or bad. I do think that all children have tremendous curiosity, and that if they have "been there, done that," they will look for new things that excite them. Those things will vary, depending on their age, but a child or, worse yet, a group of children looking for some "action" is an accident waiting to happen.

Small children may simply try to extend their world by playing in a new area. If that is the backyard of someone who has a pool, it could be big trouble. If it's in a neighboring construction site, that too could mean real danger. Even if the area is safe, you may go to find them and realize that you don't know where they are.

Children are inventive, but they could all use some help coming up with new ideas. If they are small and playing together, suggest lots of different ideas, so that if one child wants a change he or she can still have a different kind of

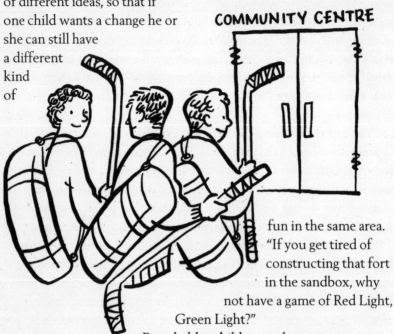

COMMUNITY CENTRE

fun in the same area. "If you get tired of constructing that fort in the sandbox, why not have a game of Red Light, Green Light?"

Bored older children and teenagers may go off looking for new territory on the transit or, worse yet, in a car. They may also look for excitement with new or different kinds of individuals whom you don't know. Both of these situations can make them very vulnerable. As a result, I believe that it's just as important to work at keeping older children and teens busy.

Many parents wait until kids have got into difficulty before suggesting that they take a part-time job, find a hobby, or get into a sport. This is a huge mistake! You'll find yourself walking up to your children and making any number of suggestions that they will say are all stupid or boring. Because they never tried the activity when they were younger, they feel that they'll make fools of themselves getting into it now. Even if they do give something a try, it takes a while to enjoy something new, and they may not have the patience to give the activity a chance. Consequently, it's important that you get your children involved in activities when they are still very young. It's also important to let your children do or play at something that interests them, not just you.

Beginning when they were five years old, I tried getting my children to participate in soccer. There are endless house leagues that emphasize participation rather than competition. Two of my kids showed a real interest and have kept it up into their teenage years through competitive leagues. The other two tried soccer for a season. I wanted them to stay with it long enough to give it a real chance before they decided they'd rather have a go at something else. They've both become quite involved in music instead of sports.

There's no reason that kids can't participate in more than one extracurricular activity. It's true that it's going to take more involvement from you, with all of the organizing, driving, and watching involved, but that effort is a lot less onerous than a search for a missing child or dealing with a teen who has fallen in with the drug set.

There are two excellent things about keeping your children busy in organized activities. The first is that both the activities and the new friends that they meet decrease the odds of your children becoming bored. Second, as your children get better at the particular activity, it increases their self-confidence, and, as I said earlier, this is extremely important in helping them to be safe.

If you're not certain where to find things for your children to do, ask what programs are run out of the school. If none of these appeals to your children, ask other parents or go to the local community center. Such centers usually publish programs. A good idea for increasing the odds that your children will participate is to get them to join up with one or two friends. This will ease any initial shyness, and the enthusiasm of the joiner in the group will inevitably rub off on the others.

In the end, it doesn't matter what activity your children choose as long as they're doing something all year round. And remember, get them involved early.

Safety Is Everyone's Concern

Safety applies to everyone. If you make it seem like it applies only to children, then there's a huge risk that, as your children grow into their teens, they'll assume that streetproofing is only for kids and drop the good behaviors.

You can reinforce the idea that safety applies to everyone through setting a good example, which I talked about earlier. Another way is to draw your teen's attention to safety-related events that you see on the news: "Did you read about those teenagers who were in that horrible car accident?" "Yes!" "What do you think caused the driver to make that mistake?"

Discipline

There's no question that a lot of children get into trouble because they have had little discipline at home. The police tell great stories. It seems that an officer had straightened out a youngster who had been in trouble over a minor problem. Some time after, the mother called the police station. "My son won't go to bed," she said. "What shall I do?" The officer couldn't believe his ears: the woman was asking him what to do when her child wouldn't go to bed!

In another case, the officer had seen a five-year-old child utterly refuse to put on his coat when asked to do so by a parent. The mother made several threats and then gave up. She'd probably been making meaningless threats for several years. By age five, the youngster was already astute enough to recognize that he could do what he liked. His lack of respect for the adults in his immediate family had already been carried over to other adults. As the officer observed, "It doesn't matter whether the threat made in the heat of the moment is somewhat unfair; it's critically important that it's followed through."

Many parents have forgotten that they have rights, including the right to discipline their children. A great number of parents are now being pushed around by their kids, something almost inconceivable only a generation ago.

The police agree unanimously that, with rare exceptions, parents know what is best for their children. It seems ludicrous to them that the people who live with a child would want advice from a police officer whose contact with the youngster probably lasted less than a day. Kids should have greater respect for information from their parents. The police believe that if parents would simply trust their own judgment, and exercise their rights, they'd go a long way toward helping their children.

Children Should Earn Their Privileges

Children who run into difficulties often have little sense of value. If they'd had to earn some of their privileges, they would appreciate them more. This topic circles back to parents' rights again. It is as if the effort involved in earning things when we were younger has caused us to want to give everything to our children with no strings attached. As one social worker pointed out, a child who earns an allowance even by doing something simple around the house, such as washing the dishes every other night, values the resulting privileges more and is less inclined to abuse them. In her opinion, parents have a right to expect kids to do things at home.

Social workers agree with police that today's parents must follow through on what they say. One social worker dealing with a teenage girl on probation told her that he would double her visits if she was late for a meeting without calling ahead. The girl missed an appointment and was surprised to find her reporting occasions doubled. Incredulous, she said to the social worker, "You really mean what you say, don't you?" It was quite apparent that not many people had meant what they said in that particular youngster's life.

Tips for Safety in Different Locations

1. Safety at home
★ A well-cleaned and vacuumed house is a safer house.
★ Examine the house from a child's point of view.
★ Children are always capable of more than you can imagine.

2. Home alone
★ Take the time to assess whether your child is ready to be left alone at home.
★ Ease the transition.
★ Discuss a safety checklist with your children.

3. Apartments
★ Work out safety procedures for common areas.
★ Identify safe people in the building.
★ Tell children to press the elevator alarm if they feel threatened.

4. Neighborhood
★ Walk your neighborhood to identify problem areas.
★ Discuss potential danger areas with your children.

5. Provide guidelines
★ Recognize where your children might want to go and provide guidelines.
★ Understand that your child needs his or her own space.

6. Parks and vacant lots
★ Work with local authorities to provide safe play areas.

7. Traffic
★ Kids should not count on cars obeying traffic signs.
★ The concept of death means nothing to kids under seven.

8. Shopping malls and plazas
★ Children should not go to the mall to hang out.
★ Agree on a meeting place if you and your child should become separated.
★ Point out people who could help if your child becomes lost.

9. Children and animals
★ Children should stay away from an animal unless it is with its owner.
★ If an animal is injured, children should call the humane society rather than attempting a rescue.

10. Public transit
★ Take children on public transit before they go alone.
★ Explain safety systems provided by the transit authority.

11. Changing neighborhoods
★ Make new rules for new or changing neighborhoods.

Tips for Safety in Different Locations

The purpose of this chapter is to try to help you think about the ways in which different locations affect your child's safety. It may surprise you that, according to the Canadian Safety Council, more accidents happen in and near the home than anywhere else. Consequently, this is where I'll start my discussion.

Safety at Home

Home is where your little ones spend the vast majority of their time. It's also where parents make their initial assault (especially for their first child) on making things safe. There are some excellent books on home safety. I'm simply going to mention some broad issues here.

It has always amused me how quickly I can tell, when entering a home for the first time, whether or not children live there. Inevitably, if there are small children in a home, there are no sculptures on unsteady pedestals, and nothing that can be knocked off low coffee tables.

According to Canadian statistics, the majority of childhood injuries occur in the home, particularly among young children. Not surprisingly, studies indicate that playing was the most common activity at the time the injury occurred. Two-thirds of all household injuries to children occur in the living room or the bedroom. These injuries usually happen when children lose their balance after jumping on a sofa or bed and then bump against a coffee table or dresser. Loss of balance is common among young children as their heads are disproportionately large for their bodies. As a result, falls are the most common cause of injury, although this decreases as kids grow older, while the incidence of kids being struck by objects or cut or pierced increases with age.

The most frequent time of injury is the early evening (maybe when kids are getting worn out), and substantially more injuries occur during warm or hot seasons (perhaps because of the longer days in summer, or because children are wearing more protective clothing during the winter months).

This information may prompt you to pay closer attention in some places and at some times that you may not have thought about. Obviously, playing is such an important part of learning for children that it cannot be stopped just because it involves some risk. The real point is that you must be aware of the risk and manage it as best you can.

Small children are incredibly curious and put things in their mouths. As a result, you must be conscious of every small thing within their reach. This means that a well-cleaned and vacuumed house is a safer house: no pins, nuts, stones, or buttons to swallow or put in ears or noses. However, vacuuming will not eliminate the dog's bowl or, as our family discovered to its horror, the cat's litter box.

My rule of thumb is that once children can crawl, if they can see it, they'll eventually get into it (even the kitty litter). I've got only three pieces of advice when you've got crawlers and toddlers: (1) try not to leave them alone; (2) examine the house thoroughly from a child's-eye view for potential trouble; and (3) remember that children are capable of more than you can imagine.

One day I was home alone with our first child, Patrick, who was still a toddler. I left him playing quietly on the floor in his nursery while I read the paper in the kitchen. He was absolutely quiet (a bad sign!), and when I called out to see how he was doing, he said, "Okay!" I should have known better. When finally I arrived to see how he was doing, I discovered that Patrick had put Penetan on everything within his reach. Penetan is a cream used to prevent diaper rash. It is moisture-proof and almost impossible to get off your hands, or anything else. You don't want to know how I spent the next two hours! This is when I came up with my second rule.

Get into your old clothes and literally crawl around the house on your hands and knees. Do it alone, or do it with your mate for company, but, as the Nike ads say, "Just do it!" Make sure that you go everywhere. Crawl under the dining-room table. Crawl in the basement. Crawl behind the couch. Crawl under the bed. Pull at anything that comes within reach. It's only when you've adopted your child's perspective that you'll notice what's interesting—and potentially hazardous—like the dangling light cord or the exposed springs under a bed. Everyone's home is different, and this method will provide you with a far better list of the changes that might be necessary than any book could ever come up with.

The third key thing to remind yourself of is that children are practically always capable of doing more things than you believe. As a child, I crawled out of a playpen that was on the front lawn and wandered quite a distance down our street. When a kind neighbor returned me, my astonished mother asked me how I got out. I made the mistake of showing her, and that was the end of being in the playpen on the front lawn. The moral is simple. Just because a child is not walking, you can't assume that the youngster couldn't pull a stool to a window and crawl up to look out. Rock legend Eric Clapton had a child fall from an apartment window in New York. I don't know how he or any of us could cope with such a tragedy. So, ignore the fact that your children are "too small" and take the precaution of locking the windows anyway.

As children grow older, they run and skip and wrestle without looking where they're going. As a result, they lose their balance, fall, and knock or pull things onto themselves. Rules about their indoor

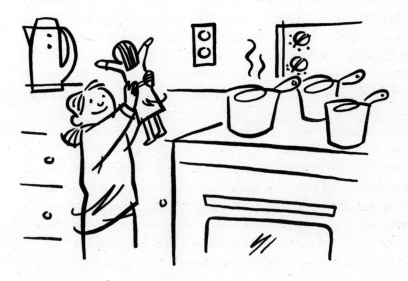

behavior are worth setting; however, they'll be broken when you are out of sight. You have three choices. Ideally, try to implement them all.

The first is to create a safe room where wild behavior is acceptable. The second is to make sure that nothing overhangs, particularly in the kitchen, where many children have been severely burned or scalded by pulling frying pans or pots onto themselves. Finally, as your children become mobile, walk them through each room and talk to them about the various things that could potentially harm them. Do it with some regularity, and ask them how they think the house could be made safer. Just as it's important for them to pay attention to their environment on the street, it's equally important for them to pay attention in the house. The problem, of course, is that it's so familiar to them that they assume it's safe, and that's when accidents happen.

Home Alone

Parents must make their own decisions as to when they feel that their children are old enough to be allowed to stay at home alone. In spite of the extremely popular Macaulay Culkin film of the early '90s, children left alone are vulnerable, and they know it. I wouldn't leave any of my children alone in the house for even half an hour until they were at least nine years old and, even then, only if the next-door neighbor was available. Crises occur in a hurry, and when they do, it's too late.

Ready or Not?

Can your children handle being left alone after school? Can you handle leaving them? To find out, take this quiz, developed by Lynette Long, Ph.D., and Thomas Long, Ed.D., authors of *The Handbook for Latchkey Children and Their Parents*. Answer each question yes or no.

1. Do you consider your child old enough to assume self-care responsibilities?

2. Do you believe your child is mature enough to care for himself?
3. Has your child indicated that he or she would be willing to try self-care?
4. Is your child able to solve problems?
5. Is your child able to communicate with adults?
6. Is your child able to complete daily tasks?
7. Is your child generally unafraid to be alone?
8. Is your child unafraid to enter your home alone?
9. Can your child unlock and lock the doors to your home unassisted?
10. Is there an adult living or working nearby that your child knows and can rely on in case of emergency?
11. Do you have adequate household security?
12. Do you consider your neighborhood safe?

If you answered no to any of the above questions, your child may not be ready for self-care, say the Longs. You should delay or abandon your plans for self-care until *all* questions elicit a positive response.

If your children want to stay at home alone, and you think they're ready, then there are some things you can do to ease the transition.

1. *Practice handling dangerous situations.* For example, have your children pretend there's a fire in each room. Ask them to tell you how the fire started, how they found it, and what they're going to do about it.
2. *Test your children.* Leave your children alone for a couple of hours. Tell them not to leave the house and to call you at a neighbor's if there's a problem. Talk to them about their experiences.
3. *Make rules that are appropriate for your children's level of maturity.* The younger the children, the simpler the rules should be.
4. *Teach parenting skills.* Younger children are frequently left in the care of older kids. Older kids need to be taught how to keep their little siblings quiet without using physical force.

5. *Consider a pet.* A pet, particularly for only children, keeps lonely feelings at bay. Caution should be exercised in selecting a breed to make sure it is compatible with children.

6. *Respect your children's fear.* Any child who's left alone is going to be afraid at one time or another. Call your children while they're alone. Come home on time. Fifteen minutes can seem an eternity to a child.

7. *Encourage your children to talk honestly about staying home alone.* Letting children talk about their fears or the way they feel can make everything right in their world.

8. *Use your guilt as a guide.* If you do feel guilty about leaving your children home alone, that's your cue to re-evaluate the situation.

Child Safety Checklist

Are your children safe when they're at home and you're at work? The National Parent–Teacher Association suggests that you make sure your children know the following things:

1. Never to go into your empty house or apartment if the door is ajar or a window broken.

2. How to unlock the door and enter an empty home. Role-play the steps to take if your child arrives home to an empty home and the door is unlocked. Be sure your child knows how to lock the door properly after entering the house and to keep the doors and windows locked.

3. How to check in with you by telephone or report to a neighbor at a regularly scheduled time.

4. How to dial the local emergency number.

5. How to get out of the house safely and quickly in case of a fire.

6. What to do if a stranger comes to the door. Pretend you are a stranger outside the front door. Remind the children not to open the door but to yell through it. Instruct them to never let a stranger know they are home alone; instead have them say that their parents are busy. Discuss your house rules on this topic.

7. How to take a phone call from a stranger. Arrange for a phone call to be made to your child. Discuss how the stranger's call was answered and how this could be improved, perhaps by teaching them to respond "My parents are busy. May I take a message?"

8. How to carry a key so it's secure but out of sight, and not to talk with friends or strangers about being home alone.

Parents should do a security check of the home before leaving children alone. Are windows safe and lockable? Are doors solid, and are the view finders low enough for a child to use them?

Apartments

Individual apartments should be treated just like a house. In addition, you must also deal with public hallways, stairways, elevators, and other common areas. The challenge with these is that they too become familiar, and therefore like home, even though they are in effect shared by all kinds of people whom you may not know.

If your children are coming home alone after school, walk them through the procedure for entering the building and the apartment. Show them where "safe" people are in the building. Discuss elevator safety. Teach your children to look confident and remain near the control panel. Let them know they can press the alarm button if they are in danger.

Neighborhood

The techniques for improving the odds for safety in your neighborhood are not much different from those for home safety. The good news is that you don't need to crawl around your neighborhood. You must, however, walk around it at a very leisurely pace—jogging will not do. If you've got a dog, walk it. If you don't, stop at the same number of posts and hydrants; that will give you a sense of the time you need to take.

If you dawdle a bit on your walk, you'll suddenly notice those locations that would make great hiding places. You'll see the spaces that exist between houses and you'll discover kids playing in a construction site that you thought was fenced off. (If this happens, I hope you'll stop and find out how they got in. Whether or not you can get those children out, you should be able to prevent an accident by discussing the dangers with your child, your neighbors, and, if you're smart, with the site supervisor.)

Provide Guidelines

Streetproofing is not a question of making a list of locations where your children cannot go. It is a recognition of where they might go. The challenge is to provide guidelines that both child and adult can accept. Let's take an example. One of the locations in your inventory of your neighborhood is a ravine. What agreement might you try to reach with your children about access to this potential hazard?

You might decide that your children can go to the ravine only when accompanied by friends during daylight hours on weekends. Before they go, have them show you the area. That means you have to go right in and walk around. You'll find that the places that would have made excellent forts when you were young are probably still being used for that purpose. Kids like to escape the adult world, and it's futile to try to stop them. However, it's nice to know where they're going.

Is the tree fort in the ravine safe? If not, the solution is not to tell your children that they can't use it. The best tactic is to explain why it isn't safe and to suggest ways to make it safer. You might even recommend tearing it down and making a new one. It's a privilege to visit your children's hideout. If you go in and destroy it, even for the best of reasons, you've probably cut off one area of communication. You simply won't hear about the next hideout. Your best bet is to go in with a genuine curiosity and interest. Tell your children about the secret places that you had when you were young. Compare yours with theirs. You'll have had tremendous success if you've located their hideout and made it a safer place to be. You'll be glad to know where your children are if you ever have to get hold of them in an emergency.

A ravine isn't the only place for a secret hideaway. Abandoned buildings are equally popular, often much more exciting, and ultimately much more hazardous. A visit to one with your children should provide you with plenty of opportunities to demonstrate why it should be an off-limits location.

Parks and Vacant Lots

Find out where the parks and vacant lots are. Even if you think you know them, wander in and examine the equipment. Is it in good shape? If it isn't, get someone to repair it, or warn your children to stay away from it. Work with local authorities to ensure your answers to the following questions regarding your children's play areas promote safety:

1. *Is there asphalt, concrete, or any other hard surface under the playground equipment?* Try to move the equipment, and if necessary, install a more resilient surface.
2. *Are buildings, paths, walkways, gates, fences, and other play areas such as sandboxes at least eight feet away from the "use zone" of each piece of playground equipment?* Your children need enough room to exit slides, jump from swings, and spin off merry-go-rounds without worrying about running into other objects or people.
3. *Are there any trees, shrubs, walls, fences, or other visual barriers that can hamper supervision of the area?* How will you know when the local clown is standing on his head on top of the climber if he can't be seen?
4. *Is there any opening that is too small to allow a child to easily withdraw his or her head?* Anything that can trap a child in any way should be removed.
5. *Do you see any sharp points, corners, or edges?* Cover the exposed ends of bolts or tubing.
6. *Are any concrete footings exposed?* Have them covered with more resilient material.
7. *Do swings bump into one another?* If so, consider removing one or two swings from a swing set.

8. *What are the swings made of?* Seats should be made of light-weight materials such as plastic, canvas, or rubber.
9. *Do the slides have protective barriers at the top?* Barriers prevent falls while your child is changing from a climbing to a sliding position, as do platforms that are at least ten inches in length.

Traffic

However your kids get to their favorite places, there's no question that they'll have to cross streets, streets that are filled with preoccupied drivers. As a result, children should be taught not to count on drivers obeying the traffic signs. The light may be red, or there may be a stop sign, but the child should be told not to step out until the vehicle has stopped.

As parents, we should realize that sometimes our kids drift off, as we do ourselves. As a matter of fact, they probably spend as much time daydreaming as they do in the real world. If you're not convinced, ask a child on the street a question. There's a reasonable chance that he or she will jump or will not hear you. Knowing that children daydream is recognizing that this altered state makes them more vulnerable. You can help your children by talking about daydreaming and pointing out situations where the inherent dangers mean that a special effort should be made to pay attention. One way of doing this is to indicate how exciting the street is. By pointing out areas of interest or how suddenly the street can change, you can help your children pay attention when they are on the street.

Pedestrian injuries are among the leading causes of death for four- to eight-year-olds and remain high through age twelve. Injuries occur when a child—perhaps obscured from the view of traffic— suddenly darts out into the street into the path of an oncoming car. Most often, mishaps occur in daylight hours on quiet residential streets close to home. In more than 25 percent of cases, the child is hit while under the supervision of a parent or other adult. It is important, then, to hold the hand of any very young child you are supervising on the street.

What about somewhat older children who play outside under

lighter supervision? Can they be counted on to stay out of the street? The answer is no. One study concluded that children typically enter the street two to ten times an hour while playing.

You need to define the boundaries of where it's safe to play by going outside and showing your children how far they're allowed to go. Draw a safe-play boundary line. Include explicit instructions for what they should do if a ball or other toy goes into the street or if another child calls to them from across the street. Make it clear they need to ask an adult for help. Talk about being a safe player and emphasize the "do's." Remember that, before the age of seven, the concept of death means absolutely nothing to a child. Dire warnings could, in fact, encourage a child to see the issue as a game: "I didn't die, so you're wrong."

Many parents tend to assume that children are safe at younger ages than is in fact the case. Children are not capable of crossing even moderately traveled streets alone until they are at least seven; they have trouble judging distances and speed. Model good pedestrian behavior. Stoop or kneel next to your child to get an idea of his or her

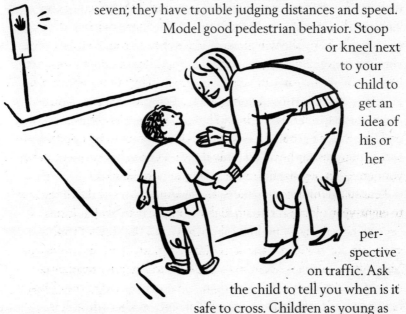

perspective on traffic. Ask the child to tell you when is it safe to cross. Children as young as two and a half can begin to learn traffic-safety habits. Teach children to make eye contact with the driver before crossing the street.

Shopping Plazas and Malls

In recent years, neighborhood shopping malls and plazas have become a significant part of many children's lives. There was no real equivalent when I was growing up. It's true that I hung out around Dot's Smoke Shop, where we bought sour grapes for a penny, but only in good weather. In the winter, when the store was standing-room only, we were chased home. Today, plazas provide warm, relatively unattended areas for kids to congregate.

Security guards at malls report disturbances created by children as young as two or three. Older youngsters tend to fool around on the escalators, often running in the opposite direction, and serious injuries have resulted. Teenagers hanging out at malls may be encouraged by the more hardened elements to try drugs. The problems are there all the time, but they are magnified after the stores close. Many malls stay open to accommodate the theater or restaurant crowd, and young people hanging around at these times are in danger of being picked up or molested. The more you talk with the security guards, the more convinced you become that, unless your youngsters are in a mall on a specific shopping trip, they shouldn't be there at all.

If you are with your children at a mall, you should agree on a place to meet if you become separated. You should then show your children how to get there, and how to identify themselves to a person in charge. Enquire if there's a supervised play area where a youngster can stay while you're shopping. If your child is going to the mall alone, provide a reasonable time limit for the trip. If he needs help, he should know who to talk to if he becomes lost: a cashier, security personnel, or a parent with a child.

Animals

A summary of a child's world would be incomplete without a knowledge of the local canine contingent. Although the breeds may vary, there's always the dog that loves every kid in the neighborhood. The animal believes it's human, goes everywhere with the gang, and licks everyone on the face. Don't ask where its tongue has been. There is also the scaredy-cat dog, usually small, that makes a terrible racket, and then runs away. Finally, there is the fierce dog, locked in someone's backyard. No danger there, right? Wrong! In our neighborhood, one of the friendliest dogs on the street was consistently teased by a group of children. One day it reached the end of its patience and, in its confusion, bit an innocent youngster. The child's stitches were out of his ankle in two weeks. By that time, man's best friend had been put to sleep. Some well-chosen words of wisdom come far too late when you've got a youngster who's terrified of animals following such an experience.

The best bet is to suggest that your children stay away from animals unless in the company of a friend who is the animal's owner. Even then, it's a better bet to leave the animal alone.

Many youngsters feel the need to come to the aid of every animal in distress, from birds through skunks. Usually the parents are not aware of the situation until the child is in distress as well. By then, the youngster may be injured or infected, and the animal is likely in worse trouble than it was before the "rescue." As soon as your child is allowed to roam the neighborhood alone, she should be instructed to call the Humane Society if she sees an animal in trouble. If for some reason she feels the animal must be moved, she should wear gloves before handling it.

Public Transit

As our children become more and more mobile at younger and younger ages, they're going to want to take public transit by themselves. The time to deal with this issue is not the day that they need to go! As a parent, you've got to anticipate this event, and take your children on the bus, streetcar, light rapid transit, train, or subway so they become familiar with public transit. Before you do this, contact the authority that runs the service and ask if they publish any safety materials. All of them have significant safety procedures in place—often far more than any of us realize—and many have employees who will go out and talk to schools and community groups. Make the

effort to find out what's available and familiarize yourself with it
before your children go off on their own. You'll find it personally helpful and reassuring. To get you started, I've included some tips from a
booklet called "Safety and Security on the TTC: A Rider's Guide,"
from the Toronto Transit Commission. Not all of these tips will apply
to your circumstances, but they will help to get you thinking.

The guide starts by emphasizing that "every employee is prepared
to help you. These employees include drivers, train guards, station
collectors, supervisory personnel, and maintenance staff. They are
easily identified by their crest."

1. **Public Telephones**

   In an emergency, you can dial 911, "0" for the operator, or the
   local emergency number from a public telephone. These meth-
   ods are always free. You will be connected with the local Police
   Emergency Center. Tell them what is happening and where
   you are. Your exact location is on a sign near each telephone.

2. **Station Collectors**

   A station collector can contact emergency personnel and give
   you information.

3. **Use "Request Stop" at Night**

   Women travelling alone can use the Request Stop program.
   - Request Stop allows a woman to get off the bus at loca-
     tions between regular stops
   - Tell the driver at least one stop ahead of where you want to
     get off. The driver must be able to stop safely in order to
     meet your request
   - Leave the bus by the front doors. The rear doors will
     remain closed so that no one can follow you from the bus

4. **Avoid Pickpockets**
   - Be alert to what's happening around you. Crowds are pop-
     ular places for the pickpocket
   - Be aware of loud arguments, bumps, or other incidents.
     They may be staged to distract you while a thief takes your
     wallet or handbag
   - Carry only what you need

- Carry your wallet in a place other than your back pocket
- If you carry a handbag, use one that closes tightly and keep it close to the front of your body

5. **Get On and Off Buses and Streetcars Safely**
   - Never run for a bus or streetcar. You may slip and fall or be hit by a vehicle
   - At streetcar stops, look before you leave the sidewalk or get off the streetcar. Make sure *all* approaching traffic has stopped
   - When boarding or leaving vehicles, keep all bags, parcels, and knapsacks clear of the doors
   - Never walk directly in front of—or behind—a stopped streetcar or bus. Other drivers may not see you
   - Never run out in front of or behind a transit vehicle. *Wait* until the bus or streetcar moves away before you step into the street so that you can clearly see other traffic

6. **Board and Exit Trains with Care**
   - While waiting on the platform, *stand back*. Stay behind the yellow safety tiles
   - When boarding or exiting the train, *mind the gap* between the train and the platform
   - When getting on subway cars, listen for the door chimes and watch for the flashing orange light in the doorway. This is a warning that the doors are about to close
   - Do not try to force open the car doors

7. **Travel Safety**
   - Never go onto the subway tracks. If you drop anything onto the tracks, get help from the station collector or any uniformed transit employee
   - Never lean against train doors
   - On buses and streetcars, never stick your arm or head out of a window

8. **In Subway Stations**
   - If possible, tell the station collector immediately about any emergency

- You can stop an escalator if someone falls or is caught. Push the red button at the top or bottom of the escalator
- Go to the nearest *Emergency Power Cut Cabinet*

9. **On a Subway**
   If a person is caught in the doors and the train starts moving, you can stop the train by using the *Emergency Stop Device*

10. **On Buses or Streetcars**
    Most buses and streetcars are equipped with a special communications system. In an emergency, drivers can call for help. They can also turn on an alarm to attract the attention of police or passers by. It's a good idea to sit at the front of a bus or streetcar to be near the driver.

No matter how many times you discuss public transit safety measures with your children, I still believe that there are two simple philosophies you should follow.

The first is, your children are always safer with one or more buddies. When they're younger, try to get them to agree to travel with an older child. When they're older, encourage them to go with a friend or, better yet, friends, and to stay together as a group when they're traveling.

Second, we all know the times when public transit is safer, and when it isn't. Common sense or a little investigation with the transit authority or the police will tell you when your children should avoid the system. Find out, and then make it a rule that they stay away during the bad times.

When the Neighborhood Changes

Many parents are aware of potential problems in their own neighborhood but make no effort to help their children if they find themselves in a new neighborhood, even for a short period of time. How many of us set new ground rules for our youngsters when we are in a new location?

Of course, parents can't know the hazards in every location, but, if they don't, they should either tour the area themselves or get together with the children and someone familiar with the new neighborhood. When youngsters are in a totally new environment, they shouldn't be allowed to go off exploring alone.

The same rule must apply to kids who are in the city for the first time. Whether they're from the country or have lived their lives in a small town or a quiet suburb, they should take special care during their first few city experiences. Youngsters unfamiliar with the number of people and the speed of the activity in the city may panic. The transit system they're traveling on for the first time may be supervised, but that will not be of help to children who aren't sure where they came from, let alone where they're going.

....

The Block Parent Program recommends that you play "What if..."games with your child. What if we get separated at the mall? What if you get lost on the way home from Billy's house? What if a group of bullies tries to steal your ball cap? Reinforce safety rules on a regular basis and give your child some alternative choices. What if there is no police officer or Block Parent to help? Where would be a safe place to get help?...a corner store, a bank, a trusted neighbor, a friend's house...Every family will have its own list of safe places.

....

To streetproof your child, you need to assume that your child knows nothing about the street. You must also recognize that the environment constantly changes. (Just as your child makes new friends and discards old ones, your neighborhood will lose some people and gain others.) Moreover, since the neighborhood will grow as your child grows, you must remain vigilant and be aware of significant changes.

Safety with People

1. **Foster a sense of community**
   ★ Teach your children how to interact with other members of your community.
   ★ Explain that they must evaluate their safety with all people.

2. **"Check first"**
   ★ Make sure your children know not to go anywhere without checking with you first.
   ★ Make sure they know not to accept anything without checking with you first.
   ★ Be careful that all your rules apply equally to everyone.

3. **Evaluate the situation**
   ★ Even well-meaning people can put your children in risky situations.
   ★ Make sure your children know it is normal to be uneasy in initial contacts with new people.

4. **Defining real friends**
   ★ Remind your children that good friendships take a long time to create.
   ★ Explain the difference between "acquaintances" and "friends."

5. **Balanced relationships**
   ★ Point out that children's friends should be similar in age.
   ★ If your children don't understand why an older person wants to be with them, they should discuss it with you.

6. **Strangers in cars**
   ★ Tell your children to stay a broom handle's length away from cars when giving directions.
   ★ Make sure your children know they should look for safe areas if a car is following them.

7. **New friends**
   ★ Instruct your children to be wary the first time they go home with a person they just know from school.
   ★ Make the effort to meet the parents of your child's friends.

8. **Sensitivity to individuals**
   ★ Children need to learn that behavior that seems normal to them may seem unusual to people from other cultures.

9. **Semi-supervised facilities**
   ★ Places like roller rinks require some basic rules of conduct.
   ★ Explain to your children that people under the influence of alcohol can be extremely unpredictable.

10. **Movie theaters**
   ★ Children should know to immediately tell an usher if unwanted advances are made.

Safety with People

As I pointed out in the introduction, child abduction is the greatest fear of all parents. While the actual number of successful abductions involving the removal of a child by a stranger for a substantial period of time or over a long distance is rather small, it can happen.

The child of a dear friend of mine in Toronto was abducted and murdered. In 1986, Alison Parrott, a promising track star, was preparing for a track meet when she was phoned and asked to go to Varsity Stadium to have her picture taken. That was the last time that she was seen alive. Through the creation of Stay Alert...Stay Safe, a non-profit national streetproofing organization, Alison's mother, Leslie, has focused her grief by helping other children avoid such a tragedy. The program offers a carefully researched range of integrated education materials, all designed to help children gain confidence in handling potentially dangerous situations and to give them the tools that can help them stay safe. The program is sponsored by Canadian Tire's Child Protection Foundation. As a member of the board of Stay Alert...Stay Safe, I am continually moved by Leslie's energy and spirit. I encourage you to make sure that your local schools and police have the Stay Alert...Stay Safe materials. Please take some time and look up the organization on the Internet at http://www.sass.ca.

Another organization was created in 1968 after a child was abducted and brutally murdered—the Block Parent Program. This national organization is non-profit, and its mission is to provide immediate assistance through a safety network as well as to offer supportive community education programs. For thirty years, in association with schools, the Block Parent Program has been educating children across Canada to keep safe. Ask your local police or school for more information about this valuable community safety program.

Although tragedies like Leslie Parrott's are extremely rare, they demonstrate that lightning can strike anywhere. In order to improve their odds of staying safe, it makes sense to take every opportunity to develop your children's skills and smarts in their interactions with people.

Foster a State of Community

Neighbors are more likely to go to each other's aid when there is a sense of community, and that sense comes from neighborhood interaction. Children must learn how to interact with and evaluate others in order to get along. They cannot learn this by being isolated. It is amazing how often so-called shy and retiring children are the ones who run into problems with others. I believe the reason is that they have not thoroughly developed their social skills.

Of all the incidents where children run into problems with adults, two-thirds involve acquaintances. Of these, one-third involve relatives. Maybe my parents' advice should have been "Don't talk to people you know, or to relatives." It sounds absurd, and of course it is, but that is in fact where the majority of big problems arise. It's not pleasant to think about, but people who want to prey on our children will often work their way into situations that put them in regular contact with young people. As a result, we must look for ideas that help children cope with the teacher, the preacher, the swim coach, and Uncle Fred.

"Check First"

At the beginning of this book, I placed a great deal of emphasis on a positive attitude. Children who are confident are less likely to be approached, abducted, or abused by sexual predators in the first place. In addition to helping children adopt this positive attitude, we need to develop some simple rules—particularly for younger children—that they can apply to everyone, whether strangers, friends, or relatives.

My favorite rule is: Don't go with anyone without checking first. Have your children check with you or your mate or, if they're at school, with the principal. The great thing about the checking rule is that it involves some time for a second opinion. It means that you as a parent have to get involved in closely examining the offer. If it's legitimate, then you can and should say yes.

The corollary to this rule is: Don't accept anything from anyone without checking first. There was a wonderful man who ran a general store near our cottage. He would occasionally offer my children free ice-cream cones. What a shame it will be if we start to feel that everyone who wants to be generous to a child is a potential pervert. The first time he was offered a cone, my son said he would have to ask me first. Sadly, the store owner was embarrassed and came to me to apologize. I knew he was a very good man, and that was confirmed in the future when he would whisper the offer to me before it was made out loud to a child whose meal might be spoiled.

The nice thing about these rules is that they make sense to young people: they apply to everyone, so you're not making anyone into a good guy or bad guy. The only time these rules are going to

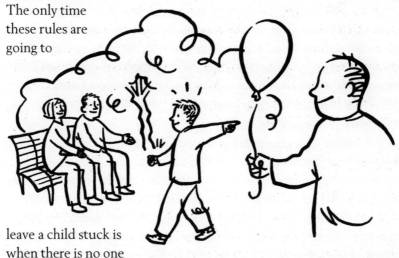

leave a child stuck is when there is no one around to consult. In cases like this, your children should know that they simply can't take up the offer.

The "check first" rule also has the benefit of opening a discussion about how decent people behave. You should talk to your children about the fact that nice people will never pressure them to respond to an invitation without allowing them time to get approval from someone in authority. You need to remind them that if an offer has to be taken up immediately, it's not an offer worth accepting. People who pressure children are in fact saying that they don't care as much about the children's needs as they do their own. If a child accepts an offer under this circumstance, he should realize that he will be pressured again and again.

Evaluate the Situation

Self-confidence is a key building block in a child's dealings with all people. While child abduction by strangers may be a parent's greatest fear, children often face their biggest risks from well-meaning adults who are caregivers. Your job as a parent is to make your children aware that they are the ones who are ultimately responsible for their own safety. If your children are participating in a supervised school or camp activity, it is up to them to carefully evaluate the situation. If they feel that there is something wrong, they must draw it to the attention of someone in authority. Depending on the circumstance, that person may or may not be accepting of the criticism. It is at times like this that your children need to know that they have your full support.

A number of years ago, a school trip was planned for a group of teenage boys. It was a canoe trip that took place in the early spring, when the water was still very cold. One morning, the group woke up next to a lake that was very rough. The staff (teachers from the school) encouraged the boys to pack the canoes and head out. No one knows what was going through the minds of those boys on that morning. As a parent, you could only hope that, if your son had been among them, he might have looked at the situation and recognized very real danger. You would pray that, realizing the risk, he might have spoken up to those in authority, dug in his heels, and said that they should wait out the weather. The teachers might have made him head out anyway. However, it is possible that, if he'd spoken up, some of the other boys might have agreed with him. It's even possible that his protest might have made one or two of the teachers reconsider their decision to move out. If this had happened on that particular spring day, a number of lives would have been saved. Sadly, it did not happen. They went out. A couple of the canoes overturned. Several boys drowned. Several staff drowned trying to save them. A tragedy was perpetrated by well-meaning adults trying to make men out of boys.

All adults have cues and signals they use to evaluate others. Discuss yours with your children. Provide them with some guidelines on how to judge the people they meet. Try to provide them with a basic understanding of what is normal behavior. For example, many people are somewhat ill-at-ease in their initial contacts with new people. Let your kids know that this is normal.

Defining Real Friends

We've all met individuals who wish to know everything about you while providing virtually no background on themselves. Kids should be taught that it's inadvisable to tell their life story to total strangers. If, in the long run, the person earns their friendship, there'll be plenty of time for swapping family histories. A person who refuses to give a little for what she gets may well be hiding a past she's not proud of. It's important to explain to a youngster that someone who is ashamed of her past should have her offer of friendship considered very carefully.

Remind your child that friendships, good friendships, take a long time to create. It is important not to send your children mixed messages on this matter. Examine your use of the word *friend*. Do you refer to people you've met only twice as "my friend"? Teach your child the difference between the words *acquaintance* and *friend*, that the people you've met just once or twice are merely acquaintances, while the people you enjoy being with and seeing regularly are your friends.

Children hear and see much more of what parents say and do than we sometimes realize, and they model their actions on the total image, not just the parts we want them to emulate. I was told a story by a friend that graphically points out the problem. My friend's wife was trying to teach their boy that the police officer was his friend, that he was a friend to the whole family and could be trusted. The only comment the little boy had was, "Well, how come he never comes to the house for drinks or dinner?" That started a whole new tack of peopleproofing—explaining the difference between acquaintances, helping friends, and personal friends. We too often ignore these differences and dump too many people into the friend category without any thought as to how it will affect our children.

Balanced Relationships

The next lesson a youngster should learn is the equal-input theorem. Your children should be taught to ask themselves what a relationship means for the other person. The best way to start the discussion is to ask them if they'd be really interested in playing with someone who is substantially younger than they are. If they look at you as though they think you've lost your mind, then raise the reverse possibility. What would they think if someone substantially older wanted to spend a great deal of time in their company? The general point is that children of similar ages usually have similar interests. If an adult is still fascinated by what kids are up to, there may be something wrong. You can point out that there are, of course, exceptions. An older person may love telling stories to young kids. In this situation, the children learn about someone's life, and the older person has the pleasure of being valued and needed. But if an older person wants to play with your child, and your youngster can't figure out why, then he or she should discuss it with you.

People in Cars

If your seven-year-old daughter is walking along the street and a driver stops the car to ask for directions, she needs to understand that she is vulnerable. She should be alert and stay one "broom handle" away from the car. If she knows the directions, she's welcome to provide a polite answer. However, if the driver asks to be taken to the location, she should refuse the request. If you walk children through this scenario, it makes more sense to them than a blanket statement such as "Don't talk to strangers." As a result, they're more likely to take you seriously.

Discuss appropriate responses to a variety of situations. For example, if your child is walking along a street and a car slows down to follow her, she should double back and walk in the opposite direction. If the car turns to follow her, she should run to the nearest safe location and report the incident. If, on the other hand, an unknown woman asks a group of four fifteen-year-olds to help her change a tire, they should help.

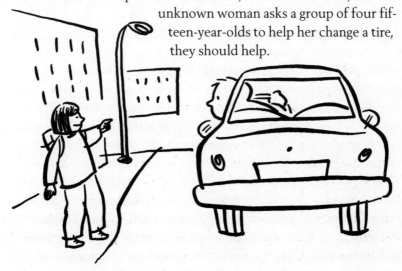

As you travel the streets with your children, play the game "Would You Do This?" By creating various situations, you can help them appreciate when they are more and less vulnerable and, as a result, when they should be more on their guard.

New Friends

Unfortunately, children's vulnerability is not limited to strangers in cars. It also exists when children encounter a person they know in a new environment. Children should be wary the first time they go to the home of a person they just know from school. When I was young, I met another young boy at school. The first time I went to his house, I was shocked to find that he owned a bullwhip, which he proceeded to flick dangerously close to my face. I was genuinely frightened and, although the event did not result in injury, I avoided being alone with the boy from then on.

A friend of ours related a similar experience. As a teenager, he visited a very popular teacher at his home. In retrospect he knew he was lucky not to have been confronted with a sexual advance. Again, the facts are simple: people are not always the same in one environment as they are in another.

The best way to avoid this kind of unpleasant situation is to make an effort to meet your child's friends and parents. It doesn't have to be an unpleasant task. As a matter of fact, it can be a great deal of fun. Do you know what your kid's friends like to do? Do you know the places where they meet with each other? Who's the guy or girl whose opinions mean the most to the rest of the group? You'll want to size that person up. If it's your own child, you're faced with some pretty specific questions. Only by knowing the neighborhood chums can you appreciate the kinds of pressures that your child is under. Only by understanding how these children think can you have an insight into how your suggestions are being evaluated.

Finally, you should make every effort to get to know the parents in your neighborhood. Don't be afraid to introduce yourself and talk with them about what your kids may and may not do. If your children are friends of the Smith youngsters, then they'll be over at the Smiths' home. There, they'll be following Smith rules, regulations, and standards. What are Smith standards? Sometimes they're easy to figure out. After the fourth time your young child refuses dinner after playing at the Smiths' home, it should become clear that the Smiths allow their children to eat between meals.

Some kids are allowed to have friends in to play while their parents are out. If this is the case, you should know about it and make a decision as to your child's participation. Some families have power tools in the basement where the kids play. You can hope that these won't be touched, or you can do something about it. Some kids are allowed to drink wine with meals, others are not. Sometimes the differences are as simple as parents having divergent opinions as to what they'll talk about in front of their kids. We heard about a particularly popular set of parents who were a lot less reserved in front of their children. That's fine if you approve, but it should be your choice. If your youngster is spending a lot of time with a particular friend, then you should make the effort to spend an evening with the parents. They may or may not turn out to be your favorite people, but that doesn't matter. If you can get to know each other, you'll be able to place what your children are telling you in perspective.

Sensitivity to Individuals

Children need to learn that behavior that seems normal to them may be seen very differently by people from another culture. I'll give you an example. At recess one midwinter day, some young boys were involved in the usual snowball fight in a Toronto school-yard. A couple of boys newly arrived from Somalia wandered out the door, and the inevitable happened. They were pelted with snowballs.

Now put yourself in the Somali boys' shoes. They had just escaped a war-ravaged country where violence and death were everywhere. They'd barely felt their first flakes of soft falling snow, when suddenly they were hit in the head by something that felt like a rock. It's hard to imagine what they felt or thought. Even having grown up in this country, I'm still shocked when I'm caught by a snowball, so I can't imagine that they thought it was fun. At the very least, they must have thought that the intention was violent.

The next day, one of the boys showed up with a knife to take revenge. You can imagine the shock of the snowballer, trying to explain the meaning of the snowball fight when confronted by the Somali boy carrying a weapon. In war-torn Mogadishu, the boys may have felt this was the way to defended yourself. Clearly, it was an inappropriate response to a Canadian snowball fight. This was an uncommon event, the result of a war in another country. While I'm totally against snowball fights because of the risks of eye injuries and concussion, it's likely that they will continue to happen. If you allow your children to join in, tell them to make sure, before the first snowball is lobbed, that their targets are willing participants.

Semi-supervised Facilities

Semi-supervised facilities include roller rinks, spectator sporting events, and movie theaters. These places have staff on site but very little, if any, direct supervision. Your children are pretty much on their own, and therefore must be prepared to react to situations independent of adult assistance, at least until they can get someone to come to their aid.

When they're at a semi-supervised facility, your children should understand that, apart from the people they go with, they are anonymous. Once they're inside the facility, virtually no one knows they're there. For this reason, you should teach your children to follow some basic rules of conduct. To start with, your children should understand that, whenever they are in a group or a crowd of strangers, they are surrounded by a wide variety of temperaments. They have no way of knowing how any one of those strangers will react—or what will provoke a reaction. This may seem obvious on the surface, but have you ever discussed it with your child? Sometimes it's the obvious that goes unnoticed.

Caution your children never to get into an argument with a stranger. Instruct them to walk away. It's not cowardice; it's common sense. They can never know what another individual has in mind. Tell your children to report the behavior to someone in charge, change seats, or avoid the person in any way they can. If they have to leave, so be it; they won't be enjoying themselves anyway. You should tell them that, if there's the slightest doubt as to their safety, they should phone to be picked up and then wait for you in a public place.

You should also explain that people under the influence of alcohol can be extremely unpredictable. Unfortunately, at some sporting events alcohol is almost a tradition. Mixing alcohol and team support can cause some very unpleasant situations. If your youngsters find themselves sitting in front of people who are being abusive, advise them never to respond with foul or abusive language. It will serve no useful purpose and will only fuel a disagreeable situation. Caution your child never to be a peacemaker; staff and police are usually present to take on that role. Some stadiums now offer non-drinking sections. Check if this is available before your children buy their tickets.

All these suggestions apply doubly to rock concerts and rallies. You must explain that the presence of a large number of people at such events can sometimes cause individuals to behave in ways at variance with their normal behavior. At concerts, the presence of drugs adds one more dangerous element of unpredictability to what in many cases is already a frenzied atmosphere.

Movie Theaters

Because it is a darkened environment, the movie theater can be a place where unpleasantness, in the form of sexual advances, can occur. These advances can be made to boys as well as girls, and your children should be aware of that possibility. I recommend that younger children never be allowed to go to a movie, even a matinee, alone. A child sitting alone is the first target of a person intent on some covert sexual advance. Even when they're with a group, you should teach your children to move if the theater is half empty and someone comes and sits down beside them. Let them know that most people prefer to sit with as much space around them as possible. Should your child be the victim of a sexual advance, he or she should report it to an usher. Inform your child that if they are afraid to move—and that can happen—they should scream. It's better to be a little embarrassed than to be sexually molested.

Should your child be the target of unwanted sexual advances at the movies, you should go to get him and reassure him that in no way was he to blame for the incident. Do not overreact or panic. Deal with the situation openly and calmly. Much of what your child will feel about the incident will be based on his sense of your own response.

Chapter 4 Summary
Children in Charge

1. **Hiring a babysitter**
   ★ Ask for referrals.
   ★ Interview potential candidates.
   ★ Watch how they interact with your children.

2. **Leaving a babysitter in charge**
   ★ You set the rules. Don't leave it to the sitter.
   ★ Don't overburden the sitter.
   ★ Tell your children what kind of behavior you expect from a sitter—no secrets!

3. **No-tears goodbyes**
   ★ Take steps to ensure that your child will not be traumatized when it's time for you to go out.

4. **Your child as a babysitter at home**
   ★ Give it a trial run first.

   ★ Provide lots of backup help.
   ★ Come home earlier than expected.

5. **Preparing your child for babysitting away from home**
   ★ Check out the family yourself.
   ★ Provide your child with the ground rules for employment.
   ★ Inform your child that it is best to arrive early.
   ★ Consider the added factor of pets.
   ★ Make sure your child prepares by finding out about the client child in terms of temperament, adventuresomeness, and personality.
   ★ Provide guidelines if the parents come home from a party intoxicated.

Children in Charge

Hiring a Babysitter

It's important that you plan to start your search for a babysitter long before you really need one. There are always, of course, agencies you can turn to, but your best sitters will come from your neighborhood and are found by asking for recommendations from neighbors and friends who have been down the childbearing road ahead of you.

Before you start your search, establish what type of person you're looking for—age and experience, for example, and whether you have a preference for a male or female sitter. If you are new to the neighborhood, any group or organization that deals with young people is a great place to get a list of potentially responsible sitters. You may even find the same names mentioned by more than one source. The guidance department or teachers at your local high school can probably recommend a responsible person. You can also check with your local church, synagogue, community group, or Girl Guide or Boy Scout troop.

After the initial research, you can start calling your candidates. First, establish if they're interested. If they are, ask if they would be willing to come for an interview. This is critical. If they are unwilling to accept an interview, you should strike them from your list. After all, you don't want to hire anyone sight unseen. If they are willing, set an appointment that is convenient for both of you, preferably when both you and your partner can be there. You may also want to have your children present. Let them see and hear what's going on. Including your children will also give you the opportunity to evaluate the sitter's reaction to them.

Make every effort to find out all you can about the individuals you're interviewing. There are many questions you might ask. Have they taken any child care or first aid courses? Are they on any form of medication that could cause them to become drowsy or sleep too deeply to hear the children? Do they smoke? Do they have any disabilities, such as a hearing problem, that could in any way affect their performance when taking care of your children? Dr. Bryna Siegel, the author of *The Working Parents' Guide to Child Care*, suggests you ask your potential sitters how they got into babysitting, what they do to help children adjust to their parents' absence, and how they handle misbehavior.

Then watch how they interact with your child. Do they pick her up? Do they talk to her? Touch her? Does the way they talk about children jibe with the way they act toward *your* child?

And how does your child, assuming she's more than a few months old, seem to feel about the prospective sitters? You should respect your child's right not to like someone, says Dr. Siegel. She shouldn't have to put up with a babysitter she doesn't like or feel comfortable with. Nor should you.

At what age should an older child be considered responsible for the care of younger children? Twelve or thirteen is acceptable if the sitter lives next door or across the street, says Dr. Siegel, especially if his parents are available to handle any problems. Otherwise a sitter who's younger than fourteen should not be left to care for a child under three.

Family is part of a babysitter's credentials, and the quality of sitting is closely related to how interested the sitter's parents are in what their child is doing. Feel free to call the sitter's parents. Check on his experience; ask for references, especially from parents who have children the same age as your child. If your sitter is a teen, try to meet his parents. Remember, this person is a stranger to you; the more you find out about him, the less of a stranger he becomes.

Leaving a Babysitter in Charge

When you have found the person you like and, I would hope, some backup people, you might want to have him in on a day when you'll be in and out a lot. This will give you a chance to see him at work and generally get to know him better. However you want to handle it, I recommend that hard-and-fast rules be set down, rules that can be clearly understood by the sitter, the children, and yourself. There should be rules on who can come in when you're out; this should include your children's friends as well as those of the sitter. The telephone, often a source of great entertainment to sitters, should be kept free. After all, it's the only way you can get in touch should the need arise. Locking-up procedures should be clearly understood. You should also give the sitter and your children room boundaries— where they can and can't play—along with what television programs they can and cannot watch. Do this in front of your children. Let them know that the sitter is in charge while you are away. If your children are allowed to play outside before bedtime, set the curfew and lights-out time. You set the rules. Don't leave it to the sitter.

Remember, undefined areas of rules and regulations make for some very creative fibbing ("Mommy/Daddy always lets me do it"). Keep in mind that your sitter is there to watch and take care of your children, not to wash dishes, iron, or do housework. The sitter's sole responsibility should be to ensure the safety and well-being of your children in your absence.

In spite of all your precautions, it is possible to have a sitter (even one who's a relative) who demonstrates inappropriate behavior. I have a lovely niece who had an unwelcome drunken boy friend visit while she was sitting my daughter Stephanie. If some broken flower pots had not given the incident away, we might never have known. As a result, as your children get old enough to understand, it's a very good idea to involve them in an evaluation of the sitter's perfor-mance. Tell the children what kind of behavior you expect from your sitter. They could be watching for things like the sitter being on the phone all night, having friends over, or having a beer from the refrigerator. It's not your children's job to criticize the sitter, but this is information you need to know. By establishing an understanding with your children first, you've pre-empted a poor sitter's efforts to get them to keep a secret about some inappropriate behavior.

You will, of course, always want to leave numbers where you can be reached, along with your doctor's and other emergency numbers. You should also include numbers of friends, neighbors, or relatives who could assist your sitter should you be unavailable or too far away. Also show the sitter where the fuse box and flashlights are, in case of a power outage.

You will have greater peace of mind while you are away if you feel your children are in the care of a person in whom you have complete trust. But while your sitter may be competent and attentive, he may not be imaginative. So plan things to do, some games or projects for the time you are away. Remember that boredom on your children's part can lead to mischief.

No matter how much you trust your sitter, it is a good idea to take a few other precautions before you leave the house. If there are prescription drugs in your home, make sure they are locked up out of sight. The same precautions should also apply to firearms and ammunition. In short, any objects that are potentially dangerous should be safely put away under lock and key. Whether you want to believe it or not, the urge to do a little snooping can be overpowering, and no matter how well you've checked out the babysitter, there is always the possibility that curiosity will overcome better judgment.

If you require a sitter to take your children somewhere away from the home, set out the exact route they are to take. Be sure your children have proper identification as well as instructions on what to do should they become separated from the sitter. This information can be put on a card and tucked into a pocket or purse. Do not have your children wear their names on their caps!

Whatever your babysitting needs may be, bear in mind you will probably want more than one sitter. While an afternoon sitter may only be required to keep an eye on the children so you can get something done around the house, he may not be suitable to sit late at night or stay over. You may want to hire someone to walk your children to a new school for the first couple of days, but that does not mean you would trust her to take your children on a major outing. Fit the sitter to the responsibility.

One last point: Don't overburden your sitter. If you hire him, make sure he is responsible for only your children. Avoid the neighborhood leech who wants to split the babysitting tab. There are several reasons for this. First, another parent's rules may not be the same as yours, and if your children see your neighbor's kids doing something you don't approve of, it puts your sitter in an untenable position. Second, even if the rules are the same, you want your sitter's undivided attention when he is with your children. Should an emergency arise, you've compromised your emergency procedure system by adding more elements. There may be different doctors, different backup people, and possibly different locations for you and your neighbor.

I feel that if your child is in the care of a sitter, she should not have other children in the house at all, unless you are home and can personally supervise. It may seem hard-nosed, but when you think of the value of what you're placing in the trust of the sitter, you should give her every opportunity to be 100 percent attentive.

No-Tears Goodbyes

To spare the strife of tearful goodbyes when you walk out the door, psychologist Dr. Bryna Siegel recommends the following tips.

1. *Rehearse.* Leave your child for short periods of time so she begins to understand that you'll always return.
2. *Always say goodbye.* No matter how good a sleeper your child is, says Dr. Siegel, she may wake up after you've gone. If she finds a stranger in your place she'll be terrified.
3. *Keep the goodbye short.* A prolonged parting allows your child's fears about being left behind to build.
4. *Leave when your child is busy.* Separation might not look so bad when there's an interesting alternative—like Big Bird—to your presence.

Your Child as Babysitter at Home

At some point, the time will come when your child is able to stay home and look after himself and any younger siblings. The right time for this varies from family to family, but there are a number of specific precautions you can take.

The first time you leave your children alone should be a test. When you feel your youngsters are able to cope alone, give it a trial run. Don't wait until an evening when your hand is forced because you can't get a babysitter. When they're ready, pick an evening and go out for a meal at a restaurant not far from your home, or go out to visit neighbors. If there's more than one youngster, explain that there's to be no roughhousing and that no friends are to come by. They should also understand that they are not to open the door to anyone. Tell the children where you are going and leave the phone number where you can be reached. When you are at the restaurant or neighbor's house, take a break and phone home a couple of times to make sure that everything is all right. Kids will usually tell you that everything's fine, but the first time that they're left alone can be a pretty frightening experience. They'll be very glad you called. Finally, no matter when you said you'd be home—and make sure that you do specify a time—come home at least half an hour earlier. It's a good way of relieving the pressure for both you and your children, and it will provide a clear idea of what kinds of activities were taking place while you were away.

If your child clearly demonstrates to you that he is capable of staying at home alone and taking care of his siblings, then you have the first indication of whether he is capable of becoming a babysitter. Staying alone successfully is not, of course, all that's necessary for your child to take the responsibility of looking after someone else's youngster. If your child is asked to be a sitter, the very first thing you should do is give some long, hard thought to whether or not he is mature enough to take on the responsibility. There's no magic age. It's simply a question of asking yourself, would I trust my child to look after my own baby? If you feel confident that the answer to that question is yes, then your child is old enough to sit; but your responsibility doesn't end by simply giving your permission.

You should realize that if your child fails to perform his job effectively, you're going to feel responsible, whether or not the other family considers you so. As a result, it's critically important that you provide your child with the information he will require to do the job well. There are, of course, babysitting courses taught by groups such as the YMCA and the Red Cross. Even if your child has taken one of these, you can provide additional information or reinforcement about what was learned.

The first time your child is going to sit, you should have a talk with the family he will be working for. If you know the family, you can decide whether or not that particular environment is a good spot for a first experience. It should be on your child's shoulders to ask them when they expect to be in and how much they pay. Then you can both make a decision whether or not you want your child working that late. An introduction to sitting does not have to be a baptism of fire. You alone can judge whether your child's first experience would be better with a young baby, a two-year-old, or a seven-year-old.

If you don't know the family, you might ask if you could drop around briefly in order to evaluate the scene yourself. If the parents do not approve of this, you may wish to reconsider whether or not your child should sit there. As your child gains in sitting experience, he should be able to determine whether or not to work in certain homes.

Preparing Your Child for Babysitting Away from Home

It is important to explain some of the ground rules for babysitting to your child. Many, many parents are delinquent about providing this. As a result, you and your child should make up a checklist of information that should be obtained before the family goes out.

First on the list is the number at which the family may be reached. If they are at a restaurant or theater, your child should have a schedule so that she will know when to call where. The next thing that she will need to know is the name and number of a neighbor who will be in for the evening and who has been warned that he might expect a call in the event of an emergency. Naturally, it's also important to get the number of the police, the fire department, the nearest hospital, and the family doctor. The first few times your child sits, you may want to stay home yourself so she can phone you if worried.

Your child should ask if the youngster she will be minding has a routine that needs to be followed while the parents are away. Some parents forget to provide this important information, so it can't hurt to ask up front. Your child should also ask if her charge has any allergies or medical problems. Parents may not mention that a child gets asthma after he hasn't had an attack for three months.

Since sitting is often the first job experience that your child has, it gives you a good opportunity to provide her with some of the ground rules for employment. She has a right to know what she is going to be paid per hour for the evening's work. As a matter of fact, she should settle the fee on the phone before she arrives for the job. Your child should have a good indication of the hours that she'll be asked to work. Parents can't always show up exactly when they said. However, they should be within half an hour of their predicted time of arrival or have phoned with a good excuse. If they call and simply say, "The party's going great guns!" that should be the last evening your child works for that particular family. It's an unpleasant thought, but the individual hiring your child could pose a threat to her. This risk can increase if an adult has been out late drinking, and your child is staying over. The best protection you have is to check out the parents yourself. If you know them, great. If you don't, you or your child should talk to someone who does! If these precautions fail, you should discuss what she would do using the tips on self-defense from later in this book.

Arrive Early

Recommend that your child arrive ten or fifteen minutes before she is expected in order to have extra time before the parents go out. She should use this period to check out schedules and important numbers, and to find out if the house is babyproof. Most parents know what babyproofing the house means, but not all carry it through.

Your child should take time to walk very slowly through the house and examine the situation. Of course, a sitter should not leave a child unattended, but it is nonetheless important to take precautions, particularly if there is more than one child. Is there a dishwasher at floor level? Can it be latched? If it can't, are there any knives or other articles that could prove dangerous to a toddler? If there are, your child should volunteer to remove them.

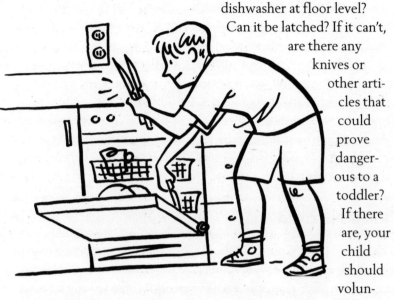

Are there cupboards that a child could open? What's in those cupboards? Is there a danger that the child could pull out a heavy object? If a room like a kitchen seems to be impossible to babyproof, possibly your child should make it out of bounds for the evening. Are there guns in the house? Silly question? Not necessarily!

Finally, if your child is sitting in an apartment, she should pay particular attention to the windows. We've all read about young children falling off apartment balconies and out of apartment windows. Usually they have pulled a stool or table over to a window so that they could stand up and look out. It's important for the sitter to make sure that all apartment doors and windows are securely locked and that stools are moved well away. If she's an inexperienced sitter, your child may not think of this particular hazard, so it's important that you discuss it with her.

Pets

The other area of concern for a sitter should be pets. The family your child is sitting for may think her particularly cautious, but she should check out Rover, the family dog, and Tigger, the family cat. The world's most lovable dogs and cats have been known on occasion to maul children. While it's often not the animal's fault—it may have been teased unmercifully—it's worth mentioning again that your child is the one who'll be responsible. Kids can often provoke a pet to its limit, and if parents aren't around to come to the rescue, it may take matters into its own paws. If your child has the slightest doubt about the situation, she should ask the parents to separate the pets and children for the evening. The fact is that they'll both survive the experience.

Know the Child

The other thing your child should do when first at a new house is pay close attention to her young charges. Are the kids climbers or explorers? Your child can ask the parents if there are any favorite hiding places in the house. Once all this has been discussed, your child should settle down and be with the younger children until they go to bed. If the parents ask your child to do odd jobs around the house, she should refuse. After all, her job is to sit, and that's enough responsibility for one evening.

It's my belief that your child should not have any visitors while sitting. If she wants to have a friend by, she should clear it with the family first. However, I believe that this practice should be discouraged. Sitting is a form of dry-land life-guarding. Similar to her counterpart at the pool, she may face long hours of inactivity. However, if a crisis occurs your child will be expected to react instantly.

If your child is sitting, you should probably leave a number where you can be reached. This will provide her with the security of knowing there's someone she trusts to consult if a questionable situation arises. In the event of an emergency, your presence may be very important.

Sleeping on the Job

If the family knows ahead of time that they are going to be very late, they may ask your child to sleep over. I advise against this, but, ultimately, you must make the decision. When you're weighing the alternatives, ask yourself if your child is a heavy sleeper. If the answer is yes, then you should discourage the idea. A friend once had a sitter who was so sound asleep that he had to break the lock on his front door in order to get into the house. Even with this noise, the sitter did not wake up until shaken by the shoulder. She was definitely not the kind of person who could have coped with a late-night emergency. If you feel that your child is capable of staying over, then you have a few more responsibilities to spell out.

First of all, he should ask his employers to wake him when they return home. Nobody needs the shock of hearing someone and wondering whether it's one of the family or an intruder. In addition, your child and the employers should establish whose responsibility the younger children are after the parents' return. If your child is to be responsible all night, then he should be rewarded accordingly, and that should be agreed upon ahead of time.

Before going to bed, your child should check that all the doors and windows are locked and that the elements in the stove have been turned off. He should also have one last peek at the child in order to ensure that nothing is amiss.

If your child is not staying over, it is the responsibility of the family to make sure that he gets home safely. If they've offered to drive your child home, you should suggest that he make sure that they're capable of driving. If he has the slightest doubt about their competence, a cab should be called. While the family should pay for the cab, you should inform your child that, if there's the slightest fuss, you'll pay. If the situation ends with a disagreement over who's paying the cab, it's probably not the spot for your child to be working anyway.

Top Safety Tips for Babysitters

When a child is given the responsibility of babysitting young children, it's important to avoid trouble spots and troubled people who could ultimately mean harm.

Stay Alert... Stay Safe offers the following tips for babysitters:

1. Avoid taking the children to lonely parks, woods, parking lots, or even schoolyards, in the late afternoon or evening.
2. When taking the children to after-school activities, always work out the best route with your employer in order to avoid unsafe places. Make sure you stick to that route each and every time. Always know where your neighborhood Block Parents are located.
3. If an adult invites you and the children you're in charge of into their home or car, always say no unless your employer has given you permission and knows exactly where you are.
4. Never open the door unless instructed to do so by your employer. Answer through a window or locked door.
5. If someone calls for your employer, tell the caller that they are too busy to come the phone right now, and take a message. Never say that they're out.
6. Make sure that there is an information and message center in every home that you babysit in. Ask your employer to leave a number where they can be reached, the children's routes home from school, their friends' phone numbers, as well as emergency numbers and procedures.
7. If you must ride on an elevator to get to and from your babysitting job, always remember to stand by the control panel in case of an emergency.
8. If someone grabs you or the children you're taking care of, scream loudly and keep screaming. Yell out "Help! Kidnap!" If screaming doesn't work, tell the child to try to spin around fast. This makes it hard for someone to hold onto them.
9. Always choose the person you want help from—a police officer, a fire fighter, a Block Parent, a teacher, a uniformed bus or subway

driver, a store clerk, or a mother or father with children. Don't allow the children to go off with anyone who approaches you to help; they might be trying to take advantage of the situation.

10. Most importantly, always pay attention to your instincts—that feeling inside that tells you something is not right. If a situation feels uncomfortable, get out of it, fast.

11. If the child has trouble breathing, and especially if he stops breathing, call for an ambulance first. Then call the neighbor and the parents, in that order. The same rules apply for poisoning or a serious fall that seems to have resulted in broken bones.

12. If the child gets a deep cut, bumps his head, or refuses to obey you, call the neighbor.

13. If the child develops a fever, begins throwing up, or won't stop crying, call the parents first.

14. Never leave the children alone. When it comes to getting into serious trouble, children are more inventive than a writer for Saturday morning cartoons.

15. Don't be afraid to ask for help. No one will think you're stupid if you have to call the parents or ask a neighbor for help or advice in handling a problem.

16. Lock the doors after the parents leave. Never open the door to strangers. Never tell visitors you're alone. If someone or something strikes you as suspicious, call the police.

17. If there is a fire, get yourself and the children out of the house quickly and safely. Don't go back into the house! Call the fire department from the safety of a neighbor's house.

Chapter 5 Summary

Team Sports and Other Supervised Activities

1. Group activities
- ★ Let your child be the one to make the decision to join.
- ★ Get to know your child's coach or leader.
- ★ Check that the personality of the activity fits with your child's.
- ★ Follow the tips provided for keeping your child safe in the world of sport.
- ★ Remember: it's only a game.

2. School excursions
- ★ Does your school have a written policy about how trips are conducted?
- ★ Use the detailed checklist for parents, leaders, students, the school and potential billeting parents.

3. Daycare and nursery schools
- ★ Check out the staff and their qualifications.
- ★ Visit the facility with your partner.
- ★ Make a follow-up surprise visit.

Team Sports and Other Supervised Activities

Participation in a physical activity with others gives children a sense of their physical capabilities. If your children are not athletically inclined, getting involved in other group activities such as Scouts, Guides, bands, cadets, parks and recreation activities, or clubs can help them learn about others, make new friends, and develop new skills.

Any activity of their choice can help build self-confidence and self-worth, which are so important to their safety and success in this world. However, these activities do put your children in a new environment which you must thoroughly check out.

Team sports occur in leagues, and I have found that different leagues have different personalities. Their personality is affected by three things: the other parents, the coaches, and whether or not the league is competitive. I'm surprised how often parents will sign up their 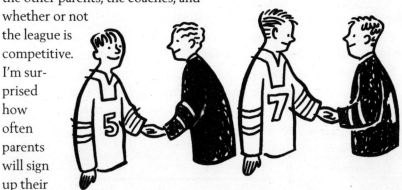 children for a league without knowing anything about its personality. It's the sport equivalent of sending their youngsters on a blind date. To my mind, it's absolutely vital that you attend a couple of games and discover the league personality for yourself. When you are there, note whether the parents applaud good plays, regardless of which side made them. Stand behind the coaches and listen to how they interact with the team. See if the children shake hands with their opponents at the end of the game. Only by doing this can you match the league's personality to your child's.

While team sports are often extremely beneficial for children, there are two factors which can make participation in sport a totally negative experience that can destroy your child's confidence and sense of self-worth. The first is a league with a bad personality. Sadly, there seem to be a lot of them.

John Bales, the president of the Coaching Association of Canada, was quoted in the *Globe and Mail* as saying, "There's enough negativism and parental pressure in the youth-sport system that we need to look very hard at how we treat children in sport." He went on to say that parents and organizers often inject pressures, frustrations, and values into children's sport that don't belong there, particularly when they emphasize winning over having fun. The seriousness of this problem is highlighted by the fact that some 70 percent of youngsters who have been introduced to organized sport drop out of it by age thirteen.

Some of the blame for this situation is attributed to the emphasis we in North America put on competition. Apparently, Europeans play down the competitive aspects of sports at young levels. In the Coaching Association of Canada's book *Straight Talk about Children and Sport*, Janet LeBlanc writes that the intensity with which many leagues approach their sport, even when it involves quite young children, means that "they've lost the sense of fun and play in sport."

I agree that children are being asked to compete too often at too young an age. Not only is this removing the fun from the sport, but, as has been documented in many sports, especially hockey, it is lowering the skill levels of the athletes who never have the time to practice new techniques.

The suggestion is often made that competitive leagues have quite different—and far more aggressive—personalities than non-competitive leagues. This does not have to be the case. As involved parents, we should be able to work toward the creation of competitive leagues where the traditions of sportsmanship and fair play are built into the code of ethics and are enforced.

The second factor that can ruin a sport is a coach who abuses the youngsters in his care. It's important to realize that abuse can include a whole range of behaviors, from emotional (constantly belittling children or calling them names) and physical (purposely slapping, kicking, or punching children, or making them do excessive exercises) to sexual (molesting children or forcing them to engage in sexual behavior). Such forms of child abuse in sports generally take place when the coach's values are not child-centered and he is more concerned with winning and fulfilling his own needs than with fulfilling the needs of the players.

Even if you have determined that your league's personality is child-friendly, you must make sure that you do a thorough investigation of the coach who is looking after your child. If you know the individual personally, this will be a great help, but you should still take the time to be around the coach when he is with your kids. It's unfortunate but true that competitive sports can bring out a side of an individual's personality and value system that you might not have seen in any other setting. The access rule is all important here. There is absolutely no reason why you shouldn't be able to visit the team (albeit discreetly) any time you want.

Volunteer coaches are, for the most part, a wonderful group who devote a great deal of their time to help kids. Still, parents have a right to know that the values espoused by the coach reflect the values the parents want to instill in their youngsters. The best way to make sure of this is for parents to get involved in the league. However, if your circumstances mean that you can't participate, and you are unhappy with what you hear, speak up. If things don't change, take your child out of that league.

Unfortunately, the problem of abuse can be far worse than a conflict over values. The conviction of Graham James, the former hockey coach of the Swift Current Broncos who pleaded guilty to two counts of sexually abusing young hockey players, serves to underline one of a parent's worst fears. It also demonstrates that the problem of abuse is not confined solely to very young children.

Stay Alert...Stay Safe published the following list of tips to help keep your kids safe in the world of sports.

1. Be your child's most important coach. Take responsibility for teaching your child what team sports are all about and what to expect. Talk about the importance of rules, cooperating with others, fair play, winning and losing, and standing up for one's rights.
2. Give your child positive feedback—always. Focus on the positives as well as correcting mistakes. Acknowledge good intentions, effort, and cooperation.
3. Encourage an open relationship with your child—establish a "no secrets" rule.
4. Make sure your kids know that what they say to you or how they feel is always more important than the sport itself or the coaches involved. In other words, make your children the center of your universe so they won't feel the need to be at the center of someone else's.
5. Let your child take part in the decision to sign up for a sport. Never force him to play a sport that he doesn't want to play.
6. Get to know your child's coach. Check up on who he is, talk to him often, and make sure he has a fair and healthy approach to his role with the children.
7. Maintain a healthy perspective yourself—and your kids will too. Remember, it's only a game.
8. More and more sports organizations now require coaches to pass police screening. The Block Parent Program suggests you check to see if this is a requirement for your child's team.

Even when your child is comfortably settled into a competitive team sport and you like and respect the coach, you still need to do some serious investigation to determine what, if any, initiation or hazing occurs. Some utterly irresponsible and tragic incidents have occurred under the guise of rites of initiation. Some have even resulted in death. The result has been a move to ban the practice of hazing altogether. Personally, I don't think that such a ban is the answer. There's more chance that initiations will be appropriate if they are monitored than if they are banned and go underground.

I think that an initiation need not be a bad thing, and in fact can be quite fun. My son Patrick played on a soccer team where the initiation consisted of him and other rookies going on what amounted to a ludicrous scavenger hunt. There was much humor about it the next day, and it brought the new team members (who had not known one another) closer together.

Coaches have a responsibility to be aware of any initiation practices. It's your job to ask the coaches about such practices and then talk to the more senior members of the team.

Any initiation or hazing should be subject to very strict rules:
- It must not involve any physical danger.
- It must not involve any degradation of the individuals.
- It must not be threatening in any way.
- It must not exploit or cause harm to anyone else in society.

School Excursions

As your children grow older, the school excursion will become more and more a part of their lives. They will pile into buses and be off for visits to provincial or state capitals, music competitions, or sporting events, and they'll be hitting the streets under the supervision of teachers and volunteers.

The first thing you should do when an excursion is announced is sit down and discuss it with your child. The initial questions— Where are you going? Who is in charge? How long will you be away?—are the easy part. Most of the information will probably be included in a notice or letter that your child will bring home from school. But don't assume that because it's a school-sponsored excursion it's immune to mishap or understaffing. It seems that all too often we have relied merely on good intentions and good luck to ensure that our children arrive safely back from these excursions.

My daughters' school had an incident when a number of girls were involved in a trip to another city. The day's activities were fine. The problems began when the group split up and the girls went to stay over with their assigned families. One of the girls went off to a suburb for dinner with her new family. After the meal, her new friend wanted to go back into the city to see a movie. The real crisis occurred when the student realized that her friend was going with a boyfriend and had a blind date for her. Her first reaction (a correct one) was to call her teacher, who was staying at a hotel in the city. Unfortunately, that was the moment

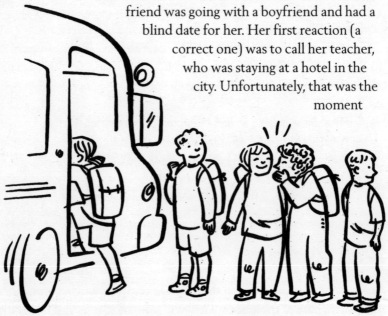

when her teacher was out having dinner. She then called home, and a very awkward situation ensued for everyone. The fallout resulted in the school setting very clear policies for such trips. In creating these, our principal attempted to get advice from other schools, only to find that very few had detailed policies in place.

Before you allow your children to participate in one of these trips, you should enquire whether their school has a written policy about how these trips are conducted, and what they would do in the case of an emergency. If your children are billeted with parents from another school, what has your school done in concert with the other school to check these parents out? What if the billet doesn't work out? For me the decision is simple: if there are no policies, or no phone, then there should be no trip.

I created the following brief summary from a very detailed field-trip procedures manual developed by Pat Parissi, the principal of St. Clement's School for girls in Toronto.

Parents should have a copy of an information permission letter which they have signed, detailing:

- dates of trip
- timetable of the day's activities
- time of departure
- mode of transportation
- names of accompanying teachers
- cell-phone number and hotel numbers at which the group leaders can be reached twenty-four hours a day

Accompanying teachers should have:

- a list of participants' emergency phone numbers
- parents' home and business numbers
- children's health card numbers
- pertinent medical information
- a cell phone
- policies for taking attendance
- written procedures should a child suffer illness, injury, or go missing
- a minimal first aid kit

Students should have:

- a clear code of conduct for while they are away (make it clear they will be sent home for bad behavior)
- a field-trip briefing
- a handout with a map, instructions, and the leaders' cell-phone number
- personal identification
- a trip "buddy"
- a code to use when calling a leader to alert him or her to a problem with a billet

The school should have:

- signed and accepted clear expectations for host parents, who must:
  - ★ have staff contact phone numbers
  - ★ chaperone and provide parental supervision for evening activities
  - ★ follow school expectations for excursions and activities
  - ★ allow visiting students to contact group leader periodically as a check
- and who must not:
  - ★ arrange any evening activity without parental supervision
  - ★ arrange activities that are not appropriate for the age levels of the students
  - ★ give any alcohol, tobacco or other restricted substances to the students

Daycare and Nursery Schools

In the case of infant or baby daycare, your child is too young to do very much to help or protect herself. You have to do it for her. I recommend that you attend the facility as an observer and walk every square inch of its property. Some daycare groups insist on it, but many don't. I also recommend that you make a surprise visit or two just to ensure that what you saw on your scheduled visit is in fact the way the facility is run on a day-to-day basis.

In conjunction with your inspection of the physical facility, check out the staff and their qualifications. Don't be satisfied with just talking to the director of the center. Remember, the director is part administrator, part public-relations manager, and part salesperson. It's not that a daycare center, whether public or private, can't have a great director as well as an efficient staff, but it's your responsibility to find out.

When I speak of checking out the staff, I mean the staff that actually interacts with the children. Check their training credentials and job experience. Talk to the dietitian; find out if she's qualified.

Determine what medical assistance is on site and what procedures are followed in the case of an emergency. Don't be afraid to ask questions. After all, it's your child, and you have the right to assure yourself that she will be taken care of in a safe manner.

The same suggestions hold true for nursery schools. Indeed, the dangers there are greater than in infant daycare because three- and four-year-olds are more mobile.

I strongly recommend that both parents go to see the facility at the same time. That way, one can do the looking while the other does the questioning. Remember that, when you're choosing a daycare center or nursery school, you're making a decision that affects your child's welfare and safety. So when you go for the interview, remember who is interviewing whom. Whatever they think of you, it's what you think of them and the facility that really counts.

Chapter 6 Summary
Victimization

1. **Strategies for avoiding abuse**
   ★ Emphasize that children should pay attention to their instincts.
   ★ Don't force children to fake affection.
   ★ Make sure your children know that physical affection is their choice.

2. **Confidence is key**
   ★ Confident children are less likely to become victims.
   ★ Confident children are less likely to be attacked in the first place.

★ Attempt to build your child's confidence.
★ Encourage your child to change passive or aggressive behavior to assertive behavior.

3. **When your child is a victim**
   ★ Make it clear the abuse was not the child's fault.
   ★ Involve all the appropriate authorities *immediately*.
   ★ Stay calm and rational.

Victimization

Who are the perpetrators of child abuse? It's not difficult for children to accept that they might face bullying in the schoolyard. It is difficult to accept, and understand, that abusers can be relatives or family members.

Strategies for Avoiding Abuse

Despite the wide range of abusers and abusive behaviors, many of the strategies for avoiding abuse apply across the spectrum. The best way to avoid victimization is for your children to try to keep themselves out of those circumstances where it might occur. As a parent, this should be your starting point.

Children should be paying attention to their instincts—those feelings that tell them that things may not be quite right. We all know that animals use their instincts to keep them alive, but modern society has confused our instincts, so we don't always use them as effectively as we could. As I said earlier in this book, following an example is very important for children, and yet instinct is an area where we don't set a very good example.

Imagine that you and your mate have just completed a very difficult week at work. You decide to have some friends over for cocktails and a leisurely dinner. The kids are flying around the house, and your baby is in the playpen, watching the action. Finally, desperate for the peace that comes when the children are tucked in, you start chasing them all to their rooms. "Time to go upstairs, guys. Come and give Uncle Harry and Aunt Margit a kiss before you go to bed." Harry and Margit aren't really an uncle and aunt, but they are close friends and have known the kids since the day they were born. Your children dutifully parade into the living room and lean toward your friends, who equally dutifully give them a peck on the cheek. Not content with this display, you pick up the baby and parade her around the room, tilting her over so that the blood runs into her head as she collects her allotment of affection. Then you pack her off to the nursery.

It all sounds quite innocent and more than a little silly. But, if you start to think about it carefully, you realize that what you're actually doing is demonstrating to your children that it doesn't matter how they feel toward someone, but rather how you feel. You are teaching them to fake affection to satisfy your own feelings for your friends. You may think this is rather innocent and harmless. However, let me fast-forward your child to a situation at summer school when she is nine years old.

She has just finished doing a lapidary project. Her teacher releases the rest of the class to the next activity and asks your daughter to stay behind for a moment because he is so pleased with the work that she has done. Flattered, your child waits. He comes up to her, and says, "I'm so proud of the work you did creating that beautiful necklace out of the stone you chose, I just wanted to give you a great big hug." Your child is aware of her instinct telling her that there is something not quite right about this person. However, conflicting with that is her experience of faking affection for adults. In an instant, a number of things go through her mind. Her desire for praise, her trust in an authority figure, and her experience with hugs from lots of adults conspire against her instincts, and she moves forward. While slightly uncomfortable, the hug is brief, and she is on her way to the next program.

No problem, right? Wrong!

If this teacher is really mixed up, then he's managed to set a precedent, a new level of accepted behavior in the relationship. There's a very good chance that he'll find another reason to be alone with your child, and a new excuse for being physically close with her. Even if your daughter's instinct is alerted, it will be even harder for her to say no because he can quite easily say, "What are you worried about? We did something like that before, and nothing happened. Aren't we special friends?" Her judgment might eventually drive her from this dangerous situation, but she could very well get in over her head because of a series of precedents that were inadvertently set many years ago with your friends.

Not for a moment do I want to suggest that physical affection isn't appropriate for your children. I am convinced that it is critically important for their balanced and healthy upbringing. I'm simply suggesting that it should be *their choice*. They're welcome to give your friends and relatives whatever affection they feel is appropriate, but if they're not in the mood, don't pressure them.

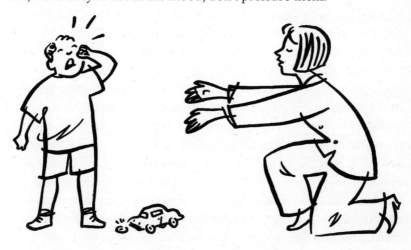

Kids feel differently about themselves and their relationships on a day-to-day basis. They may feel like hugging Granny one day and not another. My advice to my own family members is to try to move from "Come and give your old granny a hug" to having my mother open her arms and say, "Do you want to give your granny a hug?" If the response is not immediately positive, I've asked my friends and family not to pressure the child. You may have to do some explaining, but it is worthwhile. If you don't, you may be setting up a potential victim through your seemingly affectionate activities in your own home.

I'm sometimes asked about the difficulties encountered by nursery school teachers, where a reasonable dose of affection can often help a child over a mild injury or the shock of being left alone for the first time. Again, I think the solution is getting down to the child's level and offering a cuddle with open arms. If the child accepts, great. If not, the teacher shouldn't sweep over and hoist the child into the air. Instead, the teacher needs to look for another approach.

The subject of physical affection is a difficult one, and I'm the first to admit that there are a number of gray areas. Nonetheless, I think that it's better for all adults to "err on the shy side."

Confidence Is Key

Confident children are substantially less likely to become victims. This was reinforced in a study that took place at Attica, an American prison. Inmates convicted of assault and sexual abuse were asked to view a number of slides showing people of all ages and from all walks of life. They were then asked to indicate those slides that showed the people whom they were most likely to attack. Most of us would bet that they would have picked old people, particularly women, and maybe young children. On the contrary, they picked people of both sexes and all ages. These pictures were then examined by a battery of experts to see what it was that the individuals had in common.

The experts discerned three types of people among the individuals the inmates had tagged as good potential victims. The first was the awkward-looking person. People who had a disability fell into this category, but so did a young teenager who was slightly off balance because she was wearing heels that were too high. The second category consisted of people who seemed unsure of where they were going. People who were lost or who were just hanging out, the way kids do in a mall, were considered a good bet. Finally, people who looked nervous or frightened attracted the attention of the inmates.

Police have known this for years. Just as they can spot criminals from a moving cruiser, so, too, they can spot potential victims. This suggests that subconsciously they are picking up the same signals that these people are transmitting to the criminal element.

If you are trying to keep your children safe by preventing them from becoming victims, you can give some advice that will stop them from sending "attack me" signals. First, make sure that your child's clothing does not hamper her. She should wear comfortable shoes that allow her to move with ease and clothing that does not constrict her movement in any way.

Next, if your children are going somewhere, tell them to go there, do what they are going to do, and then move on. If they're going to a mall, remind them that this is an easy place for them to be observed without noticing it. Suggest that if they're going there to see a show and then afterwards go to a restaurant for a hamburger, they should do just that without hanging out anywhere in between.

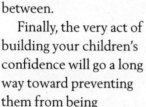

Finally, the very act of building your children's confidence will go a long way toward preventing them from being approached in the first place. If, in spite of your efforts at positive reinforcement, one of your children still seems to lack self-confidence, there are things that she can do to help herself out.

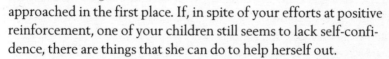

Kidscape in London, England, says that one way your child can stop being a victim is to "stop thinking like a victim." Kidscape suggests that your child do some mental exercises to build up her self-confidence. After all, "a body builder does physical exercises to build up muscles."

Your child should:
- Make a list of all the good things she can think of about herself
- Learn to talk to herself in a positive way. Instead of saying "I am so ugly no one will ever like me," say "I've got a brilliant sense of humor!"
- Develop her skill in an area in which she has a particular interest
- Think about doing something different and earning her own money; she will feel better about herself

- Do some volunteer work. Helping other people is a good way to forget about your own problems
- Find out about joining a group, whether she's interested in politics, the environment, or animal rights
- Join a youth club, religious group, or other organization
- Think about going to self-defence classes to increase her self-confidence

Victims tend to be passive. But being too aggressive can lead to trouble as well. The goal is to try to change your child's behavior from passive or aggressive to assertive. The distinctions are simple:

- Passive people behave as if other people's rights matter more than theirs
- Aggressive people behave as if their rights matter more than those of others
- Assertive people respect themselves and others equally

Assertiveness training can teach your child the different ways of responding to difficult or upsetting situations. We will touch on two important areas: making requests and saying no.

When making requests, assertive children are clear about what they want. It is important for the child to plan ahead and practice what needs to be said until she becomes comfortable. She should decide what she wants to say and stick to it: "I would like my pencil back." A request should be short and precise: "That is my pencil and I want it back."

While it sometimes may not seem that way at home, saying no is often difficult for a child. Below are some guidelines to help children say no:

- When you say no, say it firmly.
- Listen to your body and to your feelings. What do you really want to say? What do you really want to do?
- Try not to get caught up in arguments and don't become angry or upset if you don't get your own way.

- If you don't want to do something, don't give in to pressure. Be firm. Remember, you have the right to say no.
- If you are not sure and somebody is bugging you for an answer, say "I need more time to decide" or "I need more information."
- Don't make excuses: keep your body posture assertive (don't stand all hunched-up in victim mode) and look the person in the eye. The other person will know from the decisive way you are speaking and standing that you mean business. (If you find it difficult to look people in the eye, practice keeping eye contact with your family.)
- Offer an alternative: "No, I don't want to play hockey. Let's go for a walk instead." When we say no to someone, we are refusing the request; we are not rejecting the person.

Your children should be aware that if they respond to insults with more insults, the taunts can build up until they become unbearable. Your children should try "fogging" instead. When other people make hurtful remarks, the child shouldn't argue and should try not to become upset. Instead, she should imagine that she is inside a huge, white fog bank. Nothing touches her. The insults are swallowed up by the fog long before they cause her to react.

Children should learn to reply to taunts with something short and bland—"That's what you think" or "Maybe"—and then walk away. This might seem very strange at first and very hard to do, but it does work and it can help blot out insults.

Confidence and assertiveness are indispensable tools. However, they should never be a replacement for children using their common sense and instincts.

Even adults who should know better often don't use their instincts appropriately. A number of years ago, a reporter was writing about the safety of neighborhoods for an American magazine. He knew from the statistics which areas were safe, and which were potentially dangerous. While he was writing the article, he and his girlfriend went out to a movie. Parking was difficult, and so he "crossed the line," leaving his car on a street in a high-crime area. When he came out of the movie and turned up the street to pick up his car, he discovered a gang of youths hanging out by its door. His instinct said to him "Stay away." However, one of the gang members shouted to him that he simply wanted a light for his cigarette. The reporter ignored his own better judgment and approached the car. It will perhaps come as no surprise to you that he and his girlfriend were mugged by the gang. Here he was, writing an article on the subject, initially having the right inclination, and then ignoring it all and risking his life. It's an absurdly unfortunate story, but we all sometimes set ourselves up as victims.

When Your Child Is a Victim

A friend of mine has a teenage son named Ian who was shaken down for money in the restroom of a restaurant frequented by high school students. Luckily, Ian told his parents about the incident, talked to the police, and the boy went to jail.

If being a victim of a shakedown is scary for a teenager, imagine how rough things are for a child who suffers sexual abuse.

The first thing that you must make clear is that the abuse was not the child's fault. As I said at the beginning of the book, it doesn't matter how many times you've discussed safety or the need for your children to act on their instincts, your child may still find himself in an unfortunate circumstance. If this happens, you must start off by reassuring the child that nothing that occurred was his fault. Children who have been involved in even a mild case of abuse are inclined to blame themselves for not picking up on the inappropriate behavior sooner.

Next, you must involve all the appropriate authorities *immediately*. If the incident happened at school, then you should call the principal and provide her with a clear description of the situation. If it is determined that a criminal act may have occurred, and that it is necessary to involve the police or social workers, get together with them so that they all have the same information before they talk to your child. If possible, have them all together at one meeting so that your child does not have to repeat the same story a number of times.

You may find yourself having one of two quite natural reactions with your child. One might be the sweep-it-under-the-rug reaction: "It's over, sweetie... Let's not discuss it any more... Time to get on with our lives." The other is the let's-talk-it-out response: "Tell me all the details... I think you should get counseling to work this out." The fact is that most children get over most events. Your job is to listen if your child wants to talk and, if he doesn't, to move to other subjects. What he needs to know is that you are there for him, and that, if he wants outside resources, you'll provide them. Some children may find it useful to take a self-defense course to build up their self-confidence after such events.

While it is perfectly natural that you feel extremely emotional about the issue, you have to do your very best to stay calm and rational. This is the only way that you can be a real help to your child and the authorities. Remember, you have only two prime objectives. The first is to ensure that your child gets the support that he needs in order to get over the incident. The second is to make sure that justice is done and that no other children have to worry about finding themselves in the same situation with this individual again.

There's one other situation that you may come across with regard to child victimization. If you hear a rumor from your own child of another child being sexually approached by a teacher or other caregiver, you must take this information absolutely seriously, and turn it over to the authorities. Make every effort to get all the details and to corroborate the child's story. It is not good enough to say to yourself, "Well, my child is not in that class" or, worse yet, to take your child out of the school to keep him from getting into trouble. There are not a lot of bad people, but one bad person can cause a lot of harm and anguish.

Here again, it is important to stay rational and calm. If there has been inappropriate behavior, it must be dealt with. On the other hand, there have been cases where innocent people have had their lives destroyed through false accusations. Only by making sure the appropriate authorities get all the facts on both sides of the issue can you feel comfortable about having done the right thing.

Chapter 7 Summary
Bullying

1. **Types of bullying**
   ★ Bullying can be physical, racist, emotional, or sexual.

2. **Signs of bullying**
   ★ Be watchful for indications that your children are being bullied.

3. **Bullying at school**
   ★ Find out if your children's school has an anti-bullying policy.

4. **Dealing with bullying outside school**
   ★ Follow specific guidelines to deal with a bullying problem outside the school's jurisdiction.

5. **What can you do if your child is being bullied?**
   ★ Educate your children in the steps to take to handle a bully.

Bullying

Bullying is something that many of us, both male and female, experienced when we were growing up. Most of us did not cope with it well. At the very least it caused us unnecessary anguish, and in some cases it may have helped to shape negative attitudes toward others. Unfortunately, we rarely asked for help and, even if we did, society was less sophisticated then, and there wasn't really much good advice available.

When I was being picked on by another boy at school (he used to punch me continually), I finally turned to my father for help. As an ex–university-level boxer, he found the problem fairly straightforward. "The next time it happens, hit him back hard" was his advice. It did, and I did. It worked, and we ultimately became friends. However, in retrospect, I realize that it wasn't the best advice. I got away with it because I was as big as he was and he decided not to fight back. Yet it could have ended disastrously. Moreover, the advice suggested that you should try to solve a problem violently before trying to solve it through negotiation.

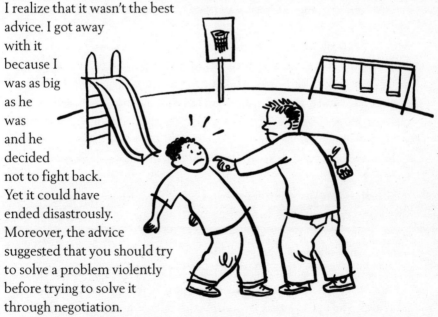

As parents, the first challenge that we face is to describe bullying clearly to children. Sometimes bullying can be very subtle, and the sooner they recognize that it's happening, the sooner they can do something about it. Bullying occurs where there is:

- deliberate hostility and aggression toward the victim
- a victim who is weaker and less powerful than the bully or bullies
- an outcome that is always painful and distressing for the victim

Types of Bullying

There are many forms of bullying. Physical bullying manifests itself in any kind of violent act. Verbal bullying includes name-calling, sarcasm, persistent teasing, and threats—"If you don't give me your dinner money, you'll be sorry." Racist bullying can be verbal as well, in the form of racial taunts, but it also includes racist graffiti or gestures. Bullying that is primarily emotional consists of deliberately excluding and tormenting the victim. Emotional bullying seems to be more common than its physical counterpart and can also be the most difficult to cope with or to prove. Finally, sexual bullying takes the form of unwanted physical contact or abusive comments.

Sexual bullying, or sexual harassment, is not the same as flirting, which is part of a mutual "getting to know you" process. Sexual harassment is unwanted attention that makes people feel uncomfortable, attacked, or humiliated. It can include taunts or touching of a sexual nature; remarks about an individual's body; suggestive or obscene letters or gestures; and derogatory posters, photographs, graffiti, or drawings.

Why do some children bully others? In some cases, children may turn to bullying as a way of coping with a difficult situation such as the death of a relative or their parents' divorce. Others are victims of abuse and take out their humiliation and anger on others. Still others want to be "top dog" and are prepared to use aggression and violence to command obedience and loyalty.

Adults who were bullied as children have a higher chance than others of acquiring a criminal record. But unchecked bullying doesn't damage just the victim. Ironically, the bully who learns that he can get away with violence is also negatively affected by his own behavior. A survey of young offenders indicated that many had been actively involved in bullying at school.

Some Myths about Bullying

"He'll just have to learn to stand up for himself." Children who tell about bullying have usually reached the end of their tether. If they could have dealt with the bullying, they would have.

"Tell him to hit back—harder." Hitting back reinforces the idea that violence and aggression are acceptable.

"That's not bullying! It's just kids teasing." Once teasing begins to hurt the victim, it is no longer "just a bit of fun" and should be stopped.

Signs of Bullying

Children may indicate by their behavior that they are being bullied. If your child shows some of the following signs, bullying may be responsible, and you might want to ask if someone is bullying or threatening him. Children who are being bullied may:

- be frightened of walking to or from school
- change their usual route
- not want to go on the school bus
- beg you to drive them to school
- be unwilling to go to school
- feel ill in the mornings
- begin being truant
- begin doing poorly in their school work
- come home regularly with clothes or books destroyed
- come home hungry (if the bully has taken their lunch money)
- become withdrawn, start stammering, show a lack of confidence
- become distressed and anxious and stop eating
- attempt or threaten suicide
- cry themselves to sleep; have nightmares
- have their possessions "go missing"
- ask for money or begin stealing money (to pay the bully)

- continually "lose" their pocket money
- refuse to say what's wrong (too frightened of the bully)
- have unexplained bruises, scratches, cuts
- begin to bully other children or siblings
- become aggressive and unreasonable
- give improbable excuses to explain any of the above

Supporting Victims of Bullying

Bullying has been compared to a form of brainwashing, with the victims ending up believing that somehow they deserved to be bullied. Victims feel vulnerable and powerless. What can you do? Keep telling your children that you love them very much and that you are completely on their side. Reassure your children that the bullying is not their fault. Explain that reacting to bullies by crying or becoming upset only encourages them.

If your children have been bullied, you may both be cheered to know that some very famous and successful people were bullied as children. Actors such as Harrison Ford, Mel Gibson, Tom Cruise, Michelle Pfeiffer, and Dudley Moore have all revealed that they were victims of bullies. All of these now famous people were "different"—which is perhaps why they were targeted by bullies—and they turned out to be more talented and successful than any of the people who bullied them.

Bullying at School

When you learn that your child is being bullied at school, keep a diary of incidents and make a note of all injuries, including photographs and details of visits to the doctor or hospital. A written record makes it easier to check facts. Keep a note of everyone you speak to about the bullying, and keep copies of any letters you write. When talking to school staff, try not to be aggressive or lose your temper. A good working relationship between you and the school should help the situation.

If the school has an anti-bullying policy, it should deal with any bullying incident in accordance with the procedures set out in the policy. These anti-bullying guidelines should be familiar to every person in the school, and pupils should understand what will happen if they persist with bullying.

The school should be prepared to:
- take the problem seriously
- investigate the incident
- interview bullies and victims separately
- interview any witnesses
- decide on appropriate action, such as:
  - ★ obtaining an apology from the bully to the victim
  - ★ imposing sanctions against the bully
  - ★ informing the bully's parents
  - ★ insisting on return of items "borrowed" or stolen
  - ★ insisting the bully compensate the victim
  - ★ holding lessons, class discussions, or assemblies about bullying
  - ★ providing a safe haven during school hours for the victim
  - ★ providing a support teacher for the victim
  - ★ encouraging the bully to change his behavior
- hold a follow-up meeting with the victim's family to report progress
- inform all members of staff about the incident and action taken
- keep a written record of the incident, interviews, and action taken

Dealing with Bullying outside School

- Keep a written record of all incidents and of all the people you talk to about the situation.
- Try to find out who is doing the bullying.
- If it is children from another school, contact their school and find out how they propose to control their behavior.

- Try having a quiet word with the bully's parents.
- Find out about local self-assertiveness courses for your child.
- Enrol your child in self-defense or martial-arts classes.
- Talk to local youth leaders who may know all the children involved.
- Inform the police.
- Video, photograph, or tape-record incidents.

What Can You Do If Your Child Is Being Bullied?

- Have your child tell a friend what is happening. Ask the friend to help you. It will be harder for the bully to pick on your child if he has a friend with him for support.
- Inform your child that he should 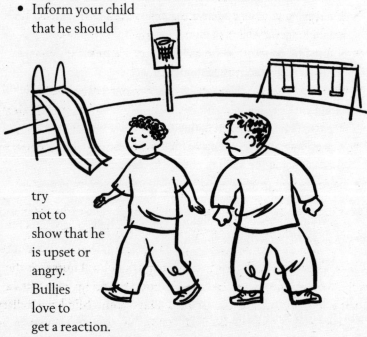 try not to show that he is upset or angry. Bullies love to get a reaction.
- Instruct your child not to fight back.
- Make sure your child understands it's not worth getting hurt to keep possessions or money. If a child feels threatened, he should give the bullies what they want.
- Teach your child not to take the bully's "bait" when the bully

first says or does something to upset your child. Reacting the way the bullies expect them to will only cause further abuse.

- Responding in a friendly manner, or with humor, will sometimes stop a bully.
- When a bully has been calling your child names, tell him that sometimes agreeing with the bully is effective—"Yeah, I know I'm a 'stupid nerd'! I sure wish I wasn't."
- Ignoring the bully by not responding and walking (not running) away can sometimes help.
- Having your child invite a bully to join a game with him and his friends is a good strategy.
- Your child should try not to brag about his possessions in front of potential bullies.
- If a bully is in your child's class, try to pick a time when he could ask for the bully's help in doing school work.
- Asking the bully about his hobbies or interests allows the bully to show pride in his world.
- If your child's strategies are not working to stop the bully's abusive behavior, make sure he tells the teacher, principal, or another adult that he trusts.
- Teach your child to walk with confidence and look people in the eye.
- Advise your child to walk and play with friends, not alone.

What if the bully is a teacher? If your child is doing his best and a teacher or other member of staff continually picks on him, humiliates him in front of others, or taunts him, then he is right to complain. Have him tell another teacher, the school nurse, or the principal what is going on. He should not cope on his own with a teacher who constantly picks on him. Have your child keep a diary of occasions when the teacher bullies him, and list the names of witnesses. Have him write down exactly what happens and how he feels.

Tips for Parents to Help Children Prevent Abduction

1. Be an attentive parent
  ★ Be particularly vigilant for young children. You are their only hope.
  ★ Teach older children:
    – the meaning of the Block Parent sign
    – to recognize suspicious behavior
    – to learn their name, age, phone number, and address

2. Pay attention to gut feelings
  ★ Make sure your children know they must act on their instincts.
  ★ Teach your children to trust their instincts, even if they turn out to be wrong.
  ★ Make sure your children learn to say no!

3. Preventing abduction attempts
  ★ Teach your children the following responses:
    – Run; possessions are not important.
    – Scream at the top of your lungs.
    – Twist and spin to get away.
    – Stay as low as possible, even becoming a "dead weight" on the ground if necessary.
  ★ Practice play-fighting with your kids.

4. Self-defense classes
  ★ Be aware that programs are effective only if:
    – they are kept up
    – the class philosophy and the teacher's is to build a child's confidence.

Tips for Parents to Help Children Prevent Abduction

In many ways, self-defense for children is what this book is all about. In spite of that, I've chosen to devote a chapter to key issues that I hope will provide a useful set of rules for helping to keep your children, or the children in your care, safe from assault or abduction.

Being a Mindful Parent

Self-protection must be handled differently, depending on the age of your child. It goes without saying that young children cannot look after themselves, and therefore their only hope is for you as a parent to keep them out of circumstances where they might get into trouble. This seems so obvious that you might wonder why I am drawing attention to it. I mention it because I've been convinced over the years that even the best of us make mistakes, and it's worth a reminder that getting away with it does not make sloppy parenting any less of a problem. We embark on our role as protector with great enthusiasm, but children are around for a long time, and all too often bad habits start to creep in.

You're in the car, heading home with your little one strapped safely into the car seat in the back. Just as you are about to pull into the driveway, you remember that you've forgotten to pick up that pound of butter you need. No problem, there's a convenience store just a couple of blocks away. It's your lucky day: you find a parking spot directly in front of the store. You open the door and realize that the temperature is dropping quickly. In your mind you analyze the pain in your lower back as you lean into the back seat to extract your daughter, who has been lulled asleep by the motion of the car. You lose your resolve and decide to lock the child in the car, saying to yourself that she will be "in view" the whole time. You know in your heart you'll only be a minute.

This scenario has happened to many of us, including me! However, we all should resolve never to let it happen again. If you take the time to think about it, you will realize that you could be engaged in conversation by someone you didn't see, or you might have difficulty finding the butter. Certainly you will take your eyes off the car for at least a few seconds—and that's all it would take. You might get away with this act a hundred times, but it's just not worth the chance. If something were to happen, you'd never forgive yourself.

Be an Attentive Parent

- Never leave your child alone in a public place, stroller, or car.
- Always accompany your child to the bathroom in a public place.
- Always accompany your child on door-to-door activities such as Hallowe'en trick-or-treating and school fund-raising efforts.
- Never leave your child unattended on your front lawn before she is old enough to know the rules of behavior for dealing with other people.

When your children are older, don't let them wander out of your direct care unless they know:

- to be alert to the people and things in their physical environment;
- their name, age, telephone number (including the area code), and address (including their street number, city, and province or state);
- how to use the phone, both with money and without money;
- the emergency response number;
- the way to get hold of you, or a designated helper, in case of an emergency;
- to tell you where they will be at all times of the day;
- what the Block Parent sign looks like, and how a Block Parent can help in times of distress;
- to carry identification;
- not to enter anyone's home without your permission;

- never to play in deserted buildings or isolated areas, or take short cuts;
- to tell you if someone has asked them to keep a secret from you.

Older children should learn to recognize suspicious behavior. They should try to remember the description of a suspicious person or vehicle and give it to you or the police. Teach them to write the plate number down as quickly as possible, even if this means using a stone on the sidewalk, a stick in the dirt, or a stick in the snow.

I have a very important word for you: Act! Police don't mind if you have made a mistake. On the positive side, they might connect your information with another detail that has been turned in, and those combined facts may make it possible for them to make an arrest. So, whether the information comes from your child or directly from you, make sure that you pass it on to the appropriate authorities.

If your children follow all of this advice, their alertness may make them aware of the potential for danger in a situation. If they sense danger, they must act immediately to *avoid the situation*. While it may not be the behavior of superheroes, your children need to be convinced that flight is better than fight. For girls, this may be a logical response. Some young boys, however, believe that all they need to do is imitate one of their television idols and everything will be all right. Explain to them that, unless they rehearse physical self-defense activities all the time, defense moves are very hard to execute. You should also point out, or even demonstrate, to them that they are not as strong as an adult, and that this puts them at a real and severe disadvantage.

Pay Attention to Gut Feelings

Children's best chance to avoid a threatening situation is to pay close attention to their instincts. The important thing to emphasize when you are discussing instinct is that there is no shame in being wrong about a hunch. Your children should be taught to act on their instinct every time, even if they find it a nuisance.

Your child is walking with a friend on the way home from school. They see an unpleasant gang of kids jostling around at the Baskin-Robbins ice cream store up the street. Your daughter's instincts make her feel a little bit uncomfortable. If she and her friend continue on the route they are following, they may be hassled. She discusses this instinct with her friend, and they decide to cut back and walk the long way home, so that they won't be seen. At home later that evening, your daughter learns that her friend's older brother was getting an ice cream, and that he would most certainly have looked out for them. Did they waste their energy taking the long route? Not at all: the trip took ten minutes longer, and, had her instincts been right, that extra time might just have kept her out of a very unpleasant situation. Why should she take the chance?

Say No

If the instinct fails, the next resort is for your child to simply and firmly say no! One evening I saw a television program in which an interviewer was talking with a child abuser who was in prison. She said to him, "If I took you out of prison and transported you to just outside a schoolyard, how long would it take you to pick up another child?" He leaned back in his chair till his face was in a shadow, and he absolutely shocked the interviewer with his answer. "About two minutes." The interviewer couldn't believe it. "Two minutes!" she said. "Yep," he answered. "And what could we do to prevent them from going with you?" she stammered. "Simply have them tell me that they won't go with me," he drawled.

In 99 percent of cases, it's that simple. The child only needs to learn to say no! Criminals are usually as lazy about the activities that they are involved in, as we can be about our own jobs. It's easier for them to find someone who will go along with them willingly than to draw attention to themselves by getting into an altercation with an unwilling victim.

Preventing Abduction Attempts

While it is extremely unlikely that your child will be abducted, it can happen. Consequently you need to have discussed his response so that it is clear what he should do. A child's first reaction should be to drop his books and his knapsack and run. Kids sometimes think they need to protect these, for fear parents will be angry if they lose them. Please tell them that their safety is more important than any possessions. The next behavior is simply to scream at the top of his lungs. He should go berserk, attempting to draw as much attention as possible to himself: "You're not my dad! Help! Kidnap!"

I know—you're reading this and thinking that you've seen a child going absolutely crazy in a supermarket where an exasperated parent was trying to get him out of the store without a handful of chocolate bars. It seemed that most people were doing their best to ignore the situation, and you're wondering if screaming really works. Well, I'm convinced that the scream let out by a child who is truly fearful for his safety is completely different from the tantrums that you'll 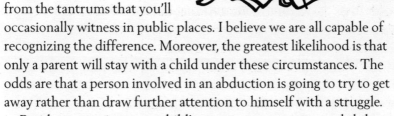 occasionally witness in public places. I believe we are all capable of recognizing the difference. Moreover, the greatest likelihood is that only a parent will stay with a child under these circumstances. The odds are that a person involved in an abduction is going to try to get away rather than draw further attention to himself with a struggle.

Besides screaming, your child's response to an attempted abduction should be to spin like a football player to try to get away. He should also stay as low as possible, throwing himself on the ground if necessary. Picking a dead weight up off the ground is a difficult proposition and may well put the attacker off balance.

Children are capable of making themselves very difficult to handle. If you've ever tried to take your younger child somewhere he didn't want to go, you will know just how difficult. The problem is that, as parents, we discourage this kind of behavior, even though there could be times when it proves very useful.

All young animals practice at play-fighting, and children are no exception. The problem is that, unless it occurs in a park, we actively discourage the behavior, worrying, quite rightly, that they might hurt themselves.

In spite of decades of discussion about the equality of women, some of us are still inclined to discourage young girls from play-fighting because their behavior may seem "unladylike." I find this strange because, if any group could benefit from the skill-set developed in mock battle, it's young girls. My bottom line is that, while you may want to carefully control the location, it is a good thing for you to play-fight with your children of either sex. Of course, they'll get the odd bump, and the prediction that "it will end in tears" will invariably seem to come true. However, I think the upsides far outweigh the downsides.

Kids hurt themselves more playing among themselves than they do wrestling with you. Providing that you don't make a fuss when they take a small bump tripping over your foot, they'll learn to carry on with a little pain, and the knowledge that they can do this may be incredibly valuable to them in later life. In addition, a good play-fight can be a terrific way of bonding with your kids. Some of the more hysterically funny moments that I've had with my children were when my youngest daughter, Stephanie, and I have taken on Caitlin and Victoria. The excited screaming and being on the bottom of the pile of kids have provided me with many fond memories. I gave up play-fighting with my son when he turned sixteen—he was starting to hurt me accidentally!

Whatever your decision about play-fighting, kids need to know that they should fight with an attacker only as a last resort. If they don't get away after screaming and spinning, they must be willing to resort to every trick in the book. They should bite, scratch, kick, knee, and do whatever it takes to free themselves.

Ultimately, the decision about allowing children to fight must be made in your family. However, given the tragic results of a number of abductions, I'd rather have my child put up a fight, and get away with some stitches or a broken bone, than go along peacefully and hope that the event will turn out to be harmless.

Whatever you teach them to do, make sure that it is instant and sudden and combined with as much hysterical noise as possible. You should also emphasize that, the moment that they break free, they must run away as quickly as possible. As soon as they are free, all the rules about safe people and safe places come into effect, and once they're safe they must tell someone all the details of the event.

Self-Defense Classes

Over the years, there has been a great deal of discussion about the benefits of martial arts, or self-defense training. Again, it has to be your decision whether the program is valuable. You should carefully check out the people giving the classes. Ideally, you should talk to parents whose children have been through the program.

I have only two cautions. First, I believe that these programs are only truly effective if they are kept up. That is, a program this year may wear off next year, and be of no value whatsoever after several years have passed. Therefore, if you're going to make the commitment, you should plan for it to be for the long term.

Second, I think these programs are beneficial only if the philosophy in the class and the instructor teaching it are both devoted to building the child's confidence. If children feel threatened or have real trouble performing the maneuvers, then such a program may sap their self-confidence, hindering their ability to stay safe.

Chapter 9 Summary

Peer Pressure

1. **"I dare you"**
   - ★ Peer pressure starts at a young age.
   - ★ Children must accept dares only when they are within their physical capabilities.

2. **Strategies to deal with peer pressure:**
   - ★ Build your child's confidence.
   - ★ Establish influence with your child's peer group.
   - ★ Keep the lines of communication open.
   - ★ Keep your children busy, for example, with responsibilities at home.
   - ★ Be willing to lose unimportant battles (like dyeing hair purple) to peers.
   - ★ Don't overreact to harmless symbols.
   - ★ Teach children the concept of consequences.
   - ★ Remember the generation gap!
   - ★ Start early: anticipate dangers, and role-play.

• •

Peer Pressure

"**P**eer pressure" is a very interesting term. When I was young, I somehow became convinced that it was a bad thing. The implication was that, if I went along with it, I would get into trouble. But peer pressure is not always a negative thing. It is nature's way of helping young adults move away from their family and grow up. Our prime concern as parents should be that they do this safely. You should initiate discussions about the issue with your children when they are quite young. In this way, you may be able to exert some influence over your children's judgment and susceptibility when they do confront peer pressure.

"I Dare You"

Peer pressure starts at a very young age with simple statements like "I dare you." The pressure from other kids can be overt, such as the dares

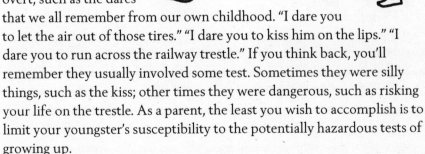

that we all remember from our own childhood. "I dare you to let the air out of those tires." "I dare you to kiss him on the lips." "I dare you to run across the railway trestle." If you think back, you'll remember they usually involved some test. Sometimes they were silly things, such as the kiss; other times they were dangerous, such as risking your life on the trestle. As a parent, the least you wish to accomplish is to limit your youngster's susceptibility to the potentially hazardous tests of growing up.

Most children haven't had much of an opportunity to prove themselves. As a result, they have to create occasions in which they can build their status. Added to this is the fact that children do not seem to have the same fears as adults. They simply haven't lived long enough to hurt themselves doing something stupid, or to see friends killed in accidents. As a result, most young people believe they're immortal.

Ask your child if she has ever been given a dare and what she thought about it. See if she can tell you why the other youngsters challenged her. The conversation should be used not as an opportunity to ridicule the dare, but to look at it as a very real part of life that your child must face. Ask if she responded to the dare, and ask whether she perceived any risk in doing so. By talking about it together, you will encourage your child to give it some thought and be better prepared to accept or reject a challenge the next time one comes along.

The other thing you can do is to tell your children stories, from news items or your own experience, in which a child runs into problems by accepting a dare. By offering examples of some of the tragedies that can occur, you can alert your youngster to potentially risky situations.

In one case, rain and inexperience proved a fatal combination for a fifteen-year-old who fell to his death down a sheer rock face near Calgary, Alberta. Reading about this tragedy, I observed that the friends who were mentioned in the article with him were both several years older than he was. Talking about the ropes that they'd hung over the edge of the cliff, one of them said, "We usually fight over who goes first, but it was raining and these cliffs were too steep. We'd only climbed some hills the week before. No one wanted to go, but suddenly Wes grabbed the rope and was over the side. He was pretty brave, and never backed down."

Although the older youths may never have thought about it, it's likely that the younger boy grabbed the rope to prove that he was a worthy partner to his friends. It's possible that he felt that he had to perform twice as well to compensate for his self-perceived inadequacies of age or size. Peer pressure works in subtle ways, and it may not always result in behavior that was what the group leaders wanted.

These "I dare you" scenarios show how important it is that you start talking about peer pressure as early as possible. If you give your children a chance to anticipate the situation and role-play in their minds, then they'll be much less subject to making a snap decision that might put them in very real danger.

Peer pressure, to most adults, is about other preteens or teens leading their poor innocent child astray. I've always wondered, if they are all poor innocent children, who is doing the leading? And where is "astray" anyway? I'm almost fifty, and I'm still not sure whether I've been there or not, but I've always thought that it might be a neat place to go. The point I'm trying to make is that we are all a bit silly about peer pressure. Your children are going to come under its influence eventually and, depending on their peers, it might be a good thing or a bad thing.

Peer pressure certainly serves a very important purpose. It helps to cut the umbilical cord that ties your children to you. You might be thinking, "How is that good?" Well, ask yourself if you still want your children around the house when they are twenty-nine years old. Some of you may think you do, but, for most of us, success in child rearing is defined as having our children out on their own, making their own way in the world.

So, peer pressure is first and foremost about children being influenced by their friends and not just by their parents. There's no point trying to fight it—you'll lose. It's better that you go along with it and try to have some influence on it.

Building Confidence

There are some very helpful strategies that you can use. The first is positive reinforcement. As has been stressed so many times in this book, confidence is key. Confident children are less likely to look to their peers to build them up. While they'll still be subject to pressure, they'll have a greater chance of saying no when they need to.

Idle Hands

If you think back to your own childhood, you'll remember that you were most subject to peer pressure when you were bored. If there's nothing better to do, you might as well go along with the gang. Right? One of the more effective ways of streetproofing your children against peer pressure is to keep them busy.

Exercise your rights as a parent and make sure that certain things are done around the home before your children are allowed to go out on the street. Such chores can include making the bed, clearing the table, feeding the cat, drying the dishes, or taking out the garbage. If children's time outside seems precious to them, they will make that time count—and hanging around is not making time count.

Influencing Your Children's Choice of Peers

The next strategy is that you can have some influence on the peer group that your child chooses. Children inevitably select their peer group from the people they meet. Ask yourself where your children meet others of their age. It seems obvious, but we often don't think about it until it's too late. When you choose where you live, you are ultimately choosing your children's peer group.

There are places where you might happily live as a childless couple. On the other hand, you might not want to raise your children there. When people think like this, they are usually thinking of safety. "Might my child be beaten up or robbed?" However, there are more critical issues. What are the children in this neighborhood like? How do they spend their time? Friends of mine lived in a very affluent community north of New York City. There was certainly little risk of crime. However, as their children became teenagers, their parents were stunned to find that the majority of teens in the neighborhood were not involved in any organized activities and spent their time doing drugs and driving around. The implication is clear. If you are going to move into an apartment or house with a new baby, and you plan to make it your home for a long time, check out what the local teens are like.

If the neighborhood is important, so is the school where you will send your children. Take the time to talk to the teachers and principal at the school your children will attend. If possible, try to meet some of the children there. Find out what they do for entertainment. Neighborhoods and schools do not change very quickly, and it'll give you an idea of whether it's an environment with which you'll be comfortable.

If you have some concerns but cannot change the school or the neighborhood, then you may want to enroll your children in some outside activities. If they are spending lots of time playing in a band or participating in a competitive sport, then there's a very real chance that those they are with will become their chosen peer group.

The Importance of Communication

Some parents try to solve the peer group issue by becoming the peer group themselves. Dads seem more inclined to do this than Moms, and I don't believe that it works. Doing things with your kids is great. The more you can interact with each child or do things as a family, the better. Parents who haven't created enough time to talk with their children often force certain answers because it's the quickest way of ending the conversation. Unfortunately, this runs counter to your efforts toward streetproofing your child. If you're going to understand what kinds of influences are being exerted outside the home, then you've got to provide regular opportunities for talking with your child. Sometimes the conversations will go nowhere. Don't worry about it. Other times you'll be provided with a genuine insight into a world that is substantially different from yours.

The most important thing is to keep the lines of communication open. You won't always approve of what you are hearing, but if your teenager is talking to you, it's a tremendous compliment, and it is generally an indication that your relationship is in good shape.

Chatting and doing things with your children does not mean you have to behave like a child. Nor does it mean that you should be their pal. You are their parent, and you love them dearly, and maybe when they are twenty-five years old you will behave more like friends. When they are children, they need you to set the ground rules. They need you to make decisions that they may not like. They need to grow up realizing that their parents have rights and responsibilities. If you're a pal, they will not be understanding and responsive to the decisions that you have to make.

Be Willing to Lose the Unimportant Battles

This does not mean that you should fight everything that your children are doing as a result of peer pressure. Your job is to evaluate the significance of the activities of the peer group and decide whether they're a natural and relatively harmless way of expressing a difference from your generation, or whether the activity actually poses a danger to your children's safety.

It's not an easy job. That's because what is normal and acceptable is changing all the time. It sounds laughable, but when I was young Beatle haircuts were enough to get teenagers sent home from school. So far, my children, both male and female, have dyed their hair purple and blonde. After the hair experiences of my youth, it didn't bother me at all. Today, there are male executives who wear earrings, and tattoos are not at all uncommon. You may not like body piercing or tattoos—I don't either. I worry about the health risks, like contracting HIV. A friend of my daughter's just had her navel pierced, and I could hardly look. My son said that he was going to get an ear pierced, and I jokingly said that I'd go along and get mine done as well. I'm not sure whether he believed me or not, but the urgency to get it done seems to have receded for a time.

Holes in the body will grow over if the ring is taken out. Tattoos are for life. A young woman who works with me has a tattoo around her wrist. She had it done as a teenager and wishes that it were no longer there. However, she has the choice of keeping it, and whatever it implies, or having a scar for the rest of her life where it was removed. My advice to my kids would be "If you've absolutely got to get a tattoo, get it somewhere where no one but your lover will ever see it." Then do a thorough check of the tattoo parlor to determine whether there is a risk of getting an infection.

Don't Overreact

As adults we've got to remember that a lot of what our children do as teens is devoted to getting a reaction. Consequently, the first rule is to avoid overreacting. If your child tells you about the kinds of activities that he is involved in, don't be too quick to disapprove. It's amazing, but kids sometimes participate in group activities even though they don't get any pleasure out of them. If this is the case, you've got an opening you can explore. After all, your goal—to make your child independent of you—is the same as that of the peer group. Tell your child that he must be his own person and take responsibility for his own actions. If the group is sneaking onto public transit without paying, then your child should understand that he, and not the group leader, is responsible for his own behavior.

Children Should Understand the Concept of Consequences

My father had a great expression: "If you're willing to accept the consequence of an activity, then go ahead and participate." Many youngsters have no sense of the consequences of their actions. They either don't realize what could happen, or they assume they can't get caught or hurt. With this in mind, it seems reasonable to ask your children if they have ever considered why they are doing certain things and what the consequences might be. It might help them to put the activity in a clearer light. If your children start to participate in some independent thinking, then they've made a major step toward independent action.

Another criterion you should encourage your children to apply to their activities is their own ability: they should engage in only those activities they can handle. If the group has decided to swim to the island and your child doesn't feel confident about making it, then he should bow out. In situations like this, your child will be able to refuse more easily if he has had lots of positive reinforcement at home and has developed a feeling of self-worth.

The analogy that I think makes the most sense out of peer pressure is that of a fast-moving stream. It's spring, and you've warned your twelve-year-old about playing near the river during the spring run-off. You are out walking the dog when you hear a splash. Your child has fallen in and is being swept downstream. As you chase him, a question flashes through your mind: "Why would he play so close to danger when we've had so many discussions about the risk?" You are panicking because you know that there is a waterfall about a kilometer downstream and you've never confronted a crisis like this.

The current is sweeping him along. You run to catch up. Your thought is to try to get him to swim back against the current, toward you. However, even if he hears your shouts and follows your directions, chances are that he'll become exhausted and slip under the water before he gets to safety.

Finally, you realize you must get him to swim with the current, cutting across it toward a point that juts out farther downstream. He risks being dragged across some rocks, but the chances are far better that he'll make it to safety, even if he is somewhat battered. After a day of rest, he will be a lot smarter and none the worse for wear.

Let me apply this analogy to some negative peer pressure. Again, you have a twelve-year-old son. The fast-moving current is the peer group. The very real danger—the swollen river—is smoking, which leads to the potentially fatal danger of the waterfall, which is lung cancer. Just as you would discuss the dangers of a swollen river, you've discussed smoking. Now, in the same way as discovering that he's fallen into the stream, you find that he's been experimenting with cigarettes.

You have two choices. You can tell him to stop instantly, that if you ever catch him with a cigarette he's grounded for a week. This is the swim-against-the-current strategy. Your second choice is to talk to him about how he might make his way with the current to that safe point. Remind him of the issues surrounding smoking. If he's involved in sports, ask him what effect he thinks smoking will have on his ability to keep up with the other players. Ask him about the financial cost of the habit and the other things that he might like to do with his money. Ask him how attractive he thinks his bad breath and stained fingers and teeth will be to potential girlfriends. You can and should mention the long-term risk of lung cancer, but you have to realize that youngsters of this age feel that they are invincible.

Cigarettes and alcohol are both difficult issues for adults and children. Children are regularly exposed to parents using both of these products. It's hard to take the moral high ground as a parent if you are not setting a good example yourself. My parents drank, but of course they were absolutely adamant that I should not. My first experience with alcohol was absolutely ludicrous. At sixteen, with the help of an older friend, I mixed gin and ginger ale and drank it on a golf course behind his cottage. The results were disastrous.

I'm now of the opinion that since children are inevitably going to try adult activities, it might make sense to allow them to do so in the safe and secure home environment. Today, there is a great deal more publicity given to the dangers of smoking and drinking than there was when I was growing up. As a result, children are more likely to be aware of the dangers of both activities. However, the fact is that example is a very strong influence. If either parent smokes or drinks, the chances are good that a child is going to want to try both at some stage.

If you've been making a strong effort to keep the lines of communication open, then you might tell your children that if, at a certain stage, they want to see what it feels like to have a smoke or drink, you'd prefer them to do it with you. The chances are good that they won't like either experience a great deal and, in your company, they won't be under any pressure to finish the bottle to be one of the gang.

Drugs

Of course, this philosophy does not work with drugs. One social worker that I talked to said that all children are going to experiment with marijuana in much the same way as our generation did with cigarettes. The solution here is obviously not to go out and purchase some so that your child can try it at home. Instead, he suggested that parents take the attitude that "the strangers who sell you that stuff are ripping you off and laughing because they've got your money." In essence, the social worker tells the kids he meets that drugs are against the law and, as a result, those people who are dealing in them are criminals. He asks them to think about what they're putting inside their bodies. Having said this, he pointed out to us that parents can't really protect kids from the drug culture. All they can do is hope that their children have enough strong values that they'll be able to place the experience in context: "I've tried it and I'm not interested."

Parties

Peer pressure and parties go hand in hand. At no other time will friends place more pressure on your child to be one of the gang. It is the last place your child will want to be different or stand out from the crowd. One thing we should remember is that adults can usually spot the opportune time to discreetly leave a party, but youngsters may not be quite as socially adept at picking the right moment to exit without a fuss from their friends. They'll be subject to "You're spoiling the party," "You're no fun," or "What a suck!" The pressure to stay is great. Consequently, the possibility of getting involved in something they don't agree with is a real problem. It's not that they're weak or that they don't have minds of their own. It's just that at a party, when the pressure's on, they're probably interested more in what their friends think of them than in what we as parents think of them.

You can do a lot to help. In the first place, you can understand what they're up against. It's no good telling them that their friends aren't really friends if they give them a hard time just because they want to leave a party or not participate in something they don't think is right. You have to give them some concrete suggestions on how to handle certain situations. One thing you should discuss with your children is the reasons they attend parties in the first place. Ostensibly it's to have fun and enjoy themselves, but if they're worried about being caught in an unpleasant situation, they should leave. If your child attends a party unaccompanied by a friend, then it is solely her decision to leave. In this situation, let her know that you are perfectly willing to come and pick her up. Assure her that there will be no inquisition, that you are willing to accept her decision to leave as proof of her ability to judge a situation and act responsibly.

If your child was driven to the party by a friend, she should ask the friend to drive her home—providing, of course, that the reason for leaving does not involve alcohol or drugs and the driver's ability is not impaired. You should also caution your child to evaluate the friend's mood before asking for the ride. If the friend is going to be angry at the inconvenience of driving her home, she is better off assuring him she can get a lift or that she'll take a cab. The last thing she will want to do is get into a car with someone who is emotionally upset.

Should the tables be turned and your child is the driver who wishes to leave the party and her friend doesn't, then she should make sure that she is not leaving her friend in the lurch, without transportation when the party's over.

Parties are a tricky problem and I'm not sure there is a standard rule, but I feel it is important to discuss the issues with your children and find out what they think should be done. After all, if the situation is such that they feel they need to get out, they should have the option to do so. The best solution I heard was from a sixteen-year-old who said she and her boyfriend always made a pact before they went to a party that, if one or the other wanted to leave, they both left. But if one wanted to stay, the person who wanted to leave could do so with no hard feelings. Very mature thinking, but I have no way of knowing whether it works. At least she seems to have thought of the possibility. Her point was that neither she nor her boyfriend liked drugs and that she would not stay anywhere they were being used. She told me that it was very hard to predict when drugs or alcohol would show up at a party, and she saw no reason to avoid all parties just because they might be used.

Your children should not be penalized for showing good judgment. No one knows what any party holds before it gets under way, so don't ground your children or forbid them to attend parties just because they came home unexpectedly early from one.

Finally, remember what it was like when you were a teen. Did you do things that drove your parents nuts? Were some of the things that you did worse than your parents knew? Remember the so-called generation gap? Now that you have children of your own, can you believe how much you end up sounding just like your parents?

Chapter 10 Summary
Where to Find Help

1. **Help for children**
   ★ Introduce your children to the police at a young age.
   ★ Educate your children about Block Parents and point out the signs.
   ★ Point out that others in uniform, e.g., transit employees, could be a help on the street.
   ★ Cell phones enable children to reach the police or an ambulance.
   ★ Make being alert a natural part of your child's routine.

2. **The information center in your home**
   ★ Include the following:
   – telephone
   – map
   – chalkboard and bulletin board
   – DayTimer
   – answering machine
   – call-waiting service

3. **Help for parents**
   ★ What constitutes an emergency?
   ★ Plan for emergencies so you can act quickly.
   ★ Lost children—a checklist on what to do, where to find help

● ●

Where to Find Help

This chapter is divided into three sections. The first is a discussion of where you should encourage your children to look for help if they find themselves in trouble. I hope to provide some useful suggestions that will make it more likely that your children will follow your advice. The second section describes how to create and use an information center in your home. Such a center can be extremely useful in the day-to-day organization of your household as well as in emergencies. The final section deals with you directly. I talk about how to identify when you need help and, more important, how to set up a process (which I hope you'll never need) to find help quickly if your child ever goes missing.

Help for Children

The Police

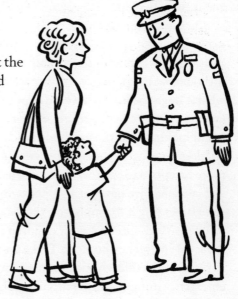

It will be no surprise to you that the first place that your child should look for help is from a police officer. You didn't need to read a child-safety book to know this. The problem is that children don't always do it. I can think of only two reasons why they don't.

The first is that we never spend enough time making police officers accessible. Think back to when you were a small child looking up at a policeman and you'll remember that the police can look rather intimidating. Today, there are even policewomen, but the uniform might still make it hard for a child to approach them. If a child is even slightly shy to begin with, he might be scared. Chances are he won't get a word out.

Sadly, your children still won't feel comfortable with the police if the example you set has not been consistent. It's no good saying "the police officer is your friend" when you're talking to your children about safety, and then cursing a traffic officer for giving you a speeding ticket. Nor is it acceptable to use the police as a threatened form of discipline with an unruly child. One police officer wrote the following letter to a newspaper to illustrate the negative side of such a practice: "When I'm in a restaurant or store with parents whose small children are misbehaving and causing a fuss, the parents will say, 'If you don't behave yourself I'm going to call that cop over here, and he will take you away and lock you up!' The parents may not realize it, but they are putting the fear of the police into the children's heads and making the law officer out to be a bad man—a person to be hated and feared. It's hard enough for us to gain the respect of children today without having this kind of image to fight. A child who is lost needs to know that the police officer is his friend, and is there to help."

You can overcome this problem while walking with your kids. When you pass a police officer, take the time to introduce your child and strike up a short conversation. When you're through, remind the kids that the police are often parents too. Talk to them about what it might be like to have a dad or a mom as a police officer. Emphasize that the police are ordinary people who have the tough job of looking after the neighborhoods where they work. Once your children have had a chance to chat with a few of them, they will be more receptive to approaching them as their first line of defense.

Even when we have set a good example about the police, we sometimes forget to emphasize the various ways they can be reached. Make sure that your children are taught how to dial 911 (or the local emergency number. There are some communities without 911, and both children and parents should know what the correct emergency numbers are). Emphasize that they can do this at a pay phone whether or not they have change. In some communities, the child does not even need to know where he is. The phone system automatically identifies the child's location. You should confirm that this is the case where you live, and then make sure that your children are aware of this exceptional feature. It can and will go a long way to ensuring a rapid and accurate response, whether they are at home alone, in a mall, or on the street.

Block Parents

Educate your child about the Block Parent Program as early as possible. For thirty years, Block Parents have been helping to make communities across Canada safer for children.

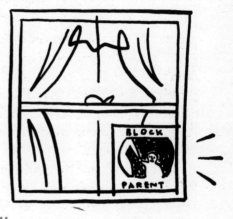

If your family resides in a Block Parent Community, walk with your child around the streets and point out homes displaying the distinctive red and white window sign. Explain to your child that the sign means there is an adult in the house who is ready to help him if he is afraid, lost, being bullied, hurt, or has been approached by a stranger to get into his car.

All Block Parents have passed a strict police screening process and there are Block Parents in every province and territory in Canada. When traveling away from your own community, should your child find himself separated from the family and in unfamiliar surroundings, he can still look to a Block Parent home for help.

If there is no Block Parent Program in your community, contact your local police and inquire about starting one. Your community will be a safer place for everyone.

Other People in Uniform

You should discuss alternatives with your children in case the police and Block Parents are not available. Approaching other people in uniform is one solution. A soldier could certainly help, but your child is substantially less likely to see a soldier than a letter carrier, crossing guard, or security guard. When you're with your children on the street, point out various individuals in uniform and talk to your children about the fact that these are people they can go to if they find themselves in difficulty.

If they're traveling on public transit, your children should also realize that the bus or subway driver or the whistle guard on a train are all people who they could count on for a quick reaction in an emergency. All transit systems have established emergency procedures for helping people. You might wish to review some of the safety tips outlined in chapter 3 with your children.

Cellular Phones

The advent of cellular phones has been a wonderful benefit to children's safety. Many cars are now equipped with phones, and a passerby can often respond to a child's cry for help by dialing for the police or an ambulance. It should be emphasized that the child needs to draw attention to himself and to be alert for vehicles equipped with car phones or radios. In urban environments, cab drivers can be a tremendous resource. Not only can they be a help themselves, but they can patch into the police and may be able to remove the child from the situation. Buses are also often radio-equipped.

Being Alert

Educating children about where they can go to be safe is a process of encouraging them to be alert to their surroundings. As they move from one neighborhood to another, children should alert themselves to who's around and where they could go for help. We all do this if we feel vulnerable. The trick is to make it a part of your child's natural routine. Where's the closest convenience store? Where are they most likely to find a lot of people? Where's the most well-lit area? Play "what if..." so you can talk to your children and see how they would react. That said, never try to determine what your children would do in a crisis by having a friend unknown to your children run a test. Child safety is about building your son or daughter's confidence, and the last thing that you want to do is create a phony crisis that may shatter all your good work.

While it's important that your children know where to look for help, it's just as important that you know when it is that your child may need assistance. Reading newspaper clippings and talking to the police has made me acutely aware of how often tragedies could have been averted if only parents had realized sooner that their children were in difficulty. Often the reason that they didn't know there was a problem is that they didn't know where their children were.

While your children will always have some time that cannot be accounted for, you can minimize that time by educating your children to be time-accountable. Time-accountability does not have to be drudgery. It can be fun, and in the long run will give them more flexibility and latitude in planning their own time and activities.

On weekdays, kids are expected to be in certain places such as school, sport practices, and so on. But, on Saturdays and Sundays, it seems that they can do as they please, and apparently many parents don't worry until it comes to spilling tears of remorse. I don't think there can be anything more frightening than being a lost child, or the parents of a lost child. The longer the child is missing, the more frightening it becomes, and the longer the odds against a safe return. With this in mind, it's just good sense to make your children time-accountable.

The Information Center

For the safety and convenience of the whole family, organize an information center in your home. It's really very simple to do and very effective. An information center is a central place in your home where members of the family leave information pertaining to their day's activities. This information should tell you or your children where any member of the family is at any given time. In this same location, all telephone numbers are kept, all emergency procedures are listed, and all appointments are recorded. In other words, whenever any member of the family needs to know where another member is, they go to the center and there's the information. The information center allows family members to communicate with each other when time and conflicting commitments don't allow for face-to-face meetings. It gives the family flexibility and at the same time demonstrates a concern for each member's well-being.

What else can an information center do for you? Well, in the case of an emergency it can cut your reaction time considerably. Because all information is centralized and recorded, there is no scrambling for phone numbers or addresses. It allows you to respond quickly by following an agreed-upon set of procedures. There is no point in a child wasting time trying to get Mommy if he knows she is between appointments, or if he knows Daddy is expected in ten minutes. In such a situation, the child could leave a message at Mommy's next destination and take whatever action the situation calls for, as listed in your emergency procedures.

The center can warn you if someone is overdue. It can also provide you with a logical and time-efficient method of locating that person, or at least with a starting point from which you can trace the person's movements.

Let's talk about the mechanics of setting up your information center and where it should be located. Since the information center consists of a number of elements, you may need to clear some space to set it up. Our information center is in the kitchen beside the phone. Yours can be in the den or family room if you prefer. It doesn't matter, provided it is located in a place the family tends to gather or pass through regularly.

Phone

The center should be near a phone and in a place where there is room to post messages and list numbers. The telephone is central to the center's efficiency. There is no use setting up a center in a place apart from the phone, as incoming messages will invariably be forgotten and not posted. So, wherever you put it, it should be near a phone.

Children should be taught from as early an age as possible how to use the phone. They should not think of it as a toy but rather as a useful and necessary piece of equipment that will help them if ever the need should arise. Of course, the young ones may not be able to read numbers, but they can be taught how to reach the operator and what to say in an emergency.

Map

While the telephone is indispensable to your center, it is only one element, especially where young children are concerned. Youngsters must be able to see what their world looks like and how the family operates. The best way to do this is by graphically illustrating it for them.

Take a walking tour of your neighborhood and draw a map of the areas where your children are allowed to play or travel. Mark the locations of the houses of your children's friends, their school, parks, and the routes they use to get to them. Now go home and, with the aid of a box of colored pencils, draw a large-scale map that can be mounted on a wall or the side of a fridge. The map is, of course, not to scale, but it starts to give your children a sense of distance and the time it takes to travel. Now your children can show you exactly where they are going and what route they intend to take. Have them show you their route before they leave. You can also mark their friends' telephone numbers right on the map. I find it is a good idea to mark my office phone number on the border of the map.

Chalkboard and Bulletin Board

Along with the map, you should mount a chalkboard and a bulletin board in your information center. The chalkboard lets you leave big, bold messages such as *"Attention—Read message on the bulletin board."* The bulletin board should have a space for every member of the family and should also have all emergency numbers (fire, doctor, hospital, police), along with numbers for your offices, clubs, and schools, as well as the makes of your cars and their license numbers. Your bulletin board is the reference book of your information center. I recommend that the whole family, not just the children, use it. If they see you using it, the board will become more meaningful for them; they will use it because you respect it. Don't let it become a repository for junk paper. It is, however, an extremely useful place to pin newspaper articles or clippings that reinforce streetproofing ideas.

DayTimer

There is one more important element you'll want to add to your information center, and that's a DayTimer, or appointment book, just like the one at the office. All appointments, club meetings, game practices, and excursions should be written down as soon as they're scheduled. You or your spouse may have to do a little probing here just to make sure the planned activity is recorded. Again, the whole family should participate. I don't think it's practical to record the events of a business day, but I do think you should record alternative numbers if you are going to be moving around and not available for long stretches of time. If it's a Saturday and both parents are running errands, you should record when you'll be returning and the general locations where you expect to be.

Other Equipment

For your older children, you may want to consider a call-waiting service. If call-waiting is unacceptable to you, then you should impose time constraints on the use of the telephone. There really isn't any need for children to conduct an hour-long conversation with someone they're going to see tomorrow or have just left fifteen minutes ago. If you teach them early in life that the phone is for messages, you shouldn't run into the problem.

If you're dealing with older children who have had unlimited use of the phone, be sure you explain why you have set new time limits. Respecting those limits is especially important when you're not home or one of the family is out and may want to check in. There is no better excuse for children being late, or not telling you they're changing plans, than "I couldn't get through—the line was busy." So the call-waiting or two-line system may be a good bet when dealing with older children.

Another piece of equipment you may want to consider is an answering machine for your phone. It's great for callers leaving messages and is available with options for leaving memos. I don't suggest that you issue your children call directors, but if you and your spouse have them, they can come in very handy when you're both out and want to check in to find out what your children are doing. They can also be very handy to give to older children when you're all going out for the day and you want to give them instructions as to where to meet you or if there's the possibility your plans might change. These machines are particularly useful if you do not have an alternative information center—that is, the number of a relative or close friend that you can leave messages with or call in the case of an emergency. This does not suggest that you should not set up your own center: it's just a backup for your family.

What if you're traveling as a family on a vacation? What can you do to keep an information center working for you while you're away? Well, for one thing, remember how valuable it is to you at home and just modify it for traveling. Set it up with new numbers at the resort or the lake. If you're visiting friends for a week and they don't have an information center, see if you can establish one in their house. The important thing is that you've got your children into an appropriate behavior pattern, and you don't want them to break that routine just because they're in a different location. Of course, you hope you'll never need your information center on vacation, but if you find yourself facing an emergency in a location that's not familiar to you, you'll be glad you took the trouble to set it up.

Help for Parents

Quick Action in an Emergency

Before I deal with what to do in an emergency, I should examine what an emergency is. Examples include a lost or injured child. It would also be considered an emergency if you were to phone home while your child is under the care of a babysitter and receive no answer. The list goes on to include children who have to cope with injured or lost friends.

You cannot possibly think of everything that could occur, but by considering what information you have about your child and his world, by playing "what if..." with yourself, and planning ahead, you can speed your reaction time. This is absolutely vital: the police and medical people alike confirm my belief that the quicker the reaction, the greater your chances of a happy ending!

However you define an emergency, there are common actions and procedures that you can follow, and that you can teach your children to follow should they find themselves in such a situation.

When Your Child Doesn't Come Home

Let's consider the worst scenario, the lost child. What do you do to recover her in the shortest time possible? The faster you establish the fact that the child is missing, the greater the chance of finding her quickly. But how do you establish that she is missing and not just dawdling or taking the long way home? If you have an information center in your home, you will check there first to make sure you haven't missed a message or misread one that tells you where she is. If there is no message or you haven't misread one, then immediately phone and check out the last place she said she'd be.

A Child Is Missing: An Action Checklist for Parents or Caregivers

- Make a careful search of your home and surrounding property.
- Check with playmates.
- Check favorite play areas.
- Call all friends, neighbors, and relatives.
- Call or visit the local police station. If you have a child identification kit, such as the one available through the Block Parent Program, take it with you. Be prepared to give the following information:
  - full physical description
  - birthmarks or other marks of identification
  - most recent photograph
  - fingerprint record card (if available)
  - description of clothing worn at time of disappearance
  - medical problems
  - recent problems at home, with playmates, and so on

- the possibility of a runaway: Are favorite clothes, possessions missing?
- the possibility of abduction by spouse or ex-spouse
- if possible abduction by parent, where the child has his or her own passport, or is recorded on the passport of the other parent

Going through a list like this at the end of the book can leave you feeling that the world's a pretty scary place. I don't believe it is!

Consequently, I'd like to finish by reminding you that the vast majority of children make it through to adulthood safely and securely. Emergencies do occur but most of them end up with a happy ending. It's amazing how many missing children are found in their own homes or at their friend's home from which they forgot to call.

As I stated at the beginning of the book, your most important job as a parent is to make your son believe in himself and give your daughter trust in her ability to take on the responsibility for her own safety with confidence. They can do it if you deal with the subject in a positive manner and make it fun. Scare tactics don't work. Lots of love and positive reinforcement will.

There's no question that it's a hard job with lots of long hours, but I firmly believe it's worth it. When you look at your own special creations going out on their own, I hope the ideas in this book will have helped you to wave goodbye with confidence, and to know that they'll be back for that wonderful family celebration with kids of their own.

References

I used several sources for the purposes of this book, some of which can serve as useful reading material. They are as follows:

A Parent's Guide to Streetproofing Children, Rick Gossage & Mel Gunton

The Handbook for Latchkey Children & Their Parents, L. Long/T. Long

The TTC Guide to Security and Safety, Toronto Transit Commission

The Working Parents' Guide to Child Care, Dr. Bryna Siegel

Straight Talk About Children & Sport, Janet LeBlanc/Coaching Association of Canada

Various booklets & pamphlets, Stay Alert…Stay Safe

And from the Internet: www.kidscape.com